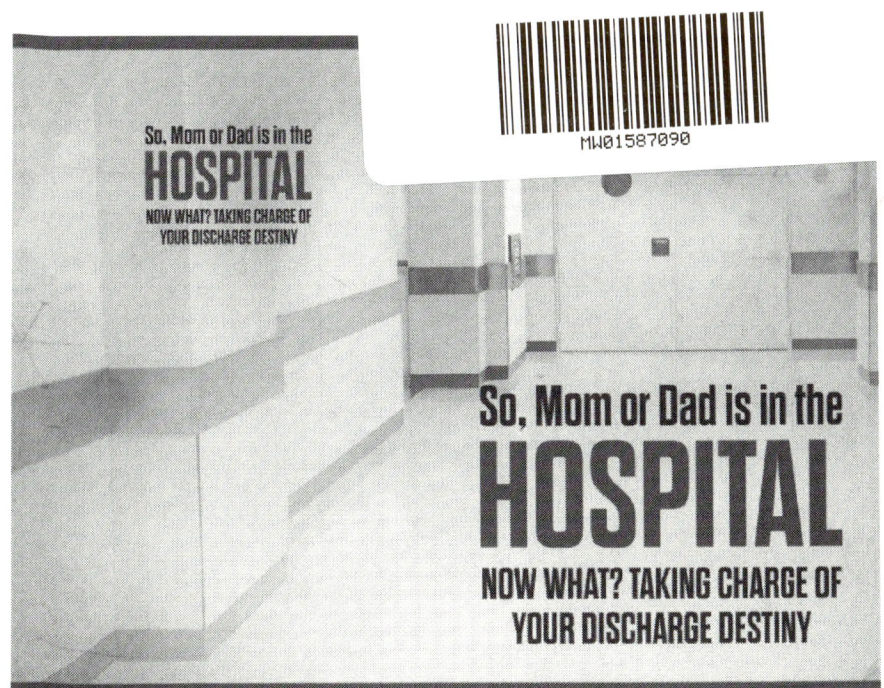

Written by our son
Robert G. Gatewood RN-ACM
"2019"

This is Dedicated to my Beautiful Wife

Christine

Thank you for all the

Love and Support

This book is intended to be a compact guide about Medicare and the important factors that are involved in the whole process from applying, claiming to qualifying for Medicare coverage. And to provide in-depth information about the concepts and processes of enrollment for you the claimant or for your mom and / or dad if the time is now, to start contemplating about extra healthcare for your parents. Finding out about your Social Security benefit entitlements and the claiming process involved with Medicare coverage may seem like difficult tasks to accomplish. This book will certainly help the reader to get a good grasp of all the factors associated with Medicare coverage, and it will keep you well informed about what can happen when you visit hospital, and / or a nursing home facility, and how it will affect your Medicare coverage.

Attitudes toward medical illnesses have changed enormously in recent years. People from all generations now expect that the treatment of even the most serious illnesses and disorders are likely to be successful. In general, people nowadays are more knowledgeable about health. When they or their children become ill, they want to know the likely cause of their symptoms and how quickly it will take for them to recover from whatever illness they are experiencing at that moment in time. We are now much more self-reliant. Most of us realize that the majority of common, and minor illnesses such as cold or an upset stomach do not need expert medical assessment or various and complex drug treatment programs to help them to recover. Those kinds of common disorders are seen as self-limiting, as we can expect to get better sooner rather than later, even if no treatment is administered by a health professional. However, the problem for many people without any medical training is that some symptoms such as a headache or an irritating cough may be the first warning sign of a more serious illness. Few events in life can be more alarming or make a parent feel more helpless than the sudden illness of their child or close loved one. Especially for a child who may be too young to describe their symptoms clearly to the parent.

But, what about the person who has parents that are currently suffering, and they do not know what to do to make them feel a little better. Or how to proceed to help them to recover, or to at least ease their pain from the constant suffering that they feel? For how long does a sensible person and/or parent deal with the problem of illness at home? When should you call a doctor or talk to an information service such as Medicare-for-you, etc? And when do you need to make an urgent appointment or to visit a hospital's accident and emergency department to help you or your parents to ease that suffering or to make a full recovery from a certain illness? What if it is mom or dad in the hospital, now what?

This book does not have all the answers to every Medicare and health question, but it is a great guide about the fundamentals of Medicare, and it will cover some of the most important aspects of mom or dad being in hospital and what to do if the worst happens and it is time for your parents to receive that much-needed extra help to try and keep them in overall good health. Understanding how the body and mind works, and how to actually look after yourself are essential if you want to stay healthy. But sadly, there may come a time, especially later in life when some people are no longer able to take care of themselves and they need outside help to keep them safe and/or to make them feel loved. Many folk in today's society have concerns about their elderly parents, and they have had to debate whether putting them in a hospital, hospice, or similar care home facilities would make mom or dad's life a whole lot easier if they did so.

But, because of its robustness, Medicare may seem a lot more complicated than it actually is. However, with the right guidance, it is not so difficult to understand the fundamental factors related to Medicare. This book will be a great guide that will help people to make an informed decision about which Medicare coverage to choose by fully understanding the Social Security system and the health coverage that is available from the government or via private companies to those in need.

Medicare coverage is currently helping more than 50 million seniors and individuals with disabilities, helping them to afford the costs of all their healthcare needs. Coverage can pay for all the patient's doctor appointments, all stays in hospital, and pay for all prescription drugs that the patient needs due to illness. The major components of Medicare and the available information for claimants in the enrollment processes will feature in this book. My aim in writing this guide is to provide a comprehensive roadmap that will outline the steps that an individual needs to take to enroll in health insurance plans and to successfully claim Medicare Benefits. The additional goal of this compact Medicare guide is to provide the reader with the comfort and the general peace of mind about their entitlements. Also, to help them find a cost-effective solution when applying for any of the available health plans and inform about the next important steps after receiving Medicare coverage.

Medicare in the United States is the federal health insurance program for people aged 65 or over, and for people aged younger than 65 years old if they are eligible by the fact that they are currently or have claimed 'Social Security Disability Insurance' (SSDI). Certain younger people who suffer from different disabilities which may need extra care that can only be provided by health professionals. If the adult and/or child has 'End Stage Renal Disease' (ESRD). They can automatically qualify for Medicare Benefit. Health coverage of this kind can be received directly through the federal government or it can be administered via a private company or a recognized medical corporation. Health insurance is a personal insurance policy that protects the individual against losses from illness. It is provided generally as regular payments and it is basically compensation for medical expenses. U.S. initiative programs like Medicare and Medicaid are mainly government-sponsored forms of health insurance, but the insurance policies can also be provided by private companies that offer individual policies, group health plans, and different plans concerning supplement insurance. Medicare Advantage Plans and Medicaid Private Drug Plans are examples of these health insurance policies that a person can apply to claim as health benefits.

Medicare eligibility for people aged under 65 years old

It is possible to qualify for Medicare before the age of 65 if you are receiving Social Security Disability Insurance, (SSDI). In most cases, the person who can qualify immediately for Medicare is usually due to a debilitating disability that may have a detrimental effect on their everyday life. Such illnesses like End-Stage Renal Disease (ESRD) – Kidney Failure - will make that person who is aged under 65 years old eligible for Medicare. However, that can depend on the individuals' current circumstances, which may include when the Medicare benefits actually started, whether the person receives dialysis in their own home or at a certain healthcare facility. And it may also have an effect on your Medicare plan if you are on the kidney transplant list at the time of claiming, or not. Eligibility can also depend on whether or not you or a loved one has paid Medicare taxes for a sufficient amount of time that has been specified by the Social Security Administration.

Medicare eligibility for people aged 65+
Medicare eligibility for the person over the aged of 65 years old is available if the individual is a U.S. citizen, and/or they have claimed or they currently qualify for the basic social security retirement benefits. People who are born outside the U.S. are still eligible if they have resided in the country as a permanent resident for five years or more. It may depend on whether you are currently receiving

the above benefit or a similar type of benefit available, like Railroad Retirement Benefit. For people who are employed or those who work on a self-employment basis, it may depend on whether they have insurance from their employer which helps them to qualify for Medicare and it's different, but associated benefits. Or, if they have contributed to a care allowance for a certain amount of time. The Medicare coverage and the number of benefits that the person receives can also depend on their work history, and how long plus how much has been paid into their Medicare contributions or health taxes beforehand.

Medicare eligibility for disabled youths under 20 years old

For parents who have a child that is under the age of 20 years old, it is possible for the child to qualify if they currently suffer from 'End-Stage Renal Disease' (ESDR). However, there are two important factors that the parent and child must be made aware of before applying to claim Medicare benefits. These factors are:

The child must need and receive dialysis on a regular basis, or the child must be on the transplant list at the time of claiming and requiring a kidney transplant.

One parent of the child must be receiving or eligible to claim Social Security retirement benefits.

If the child is 18 years old or younger and is not eligible to claim Medicare benefits, they may still be able to claim for the parents' state's 'Children's Health Insurance Program' (S-CHIP). This program is to help families who are currently considered in the low-income category. And if the child is 19 years or older, they may be eligible to claim and to qualify for Medicaid. The 'Social Security Administration' (SSA) currently judges disability, and whether the claimant actually qualifies for financial assistance basing its decision on whether or not the claimant can work.

Medicare for children aged 20+

If the child concerned in the application is over the age of 20, it is still possible for them to claim Medicare after receiving SSDI for at least 24 months. The child may also be able to claim and qualify for SSDI, even if they have had no past work history, but there are certain factors to be aware of for the insurance claim to be successful:

The child must have developed the disability before the age of 22 years old.

They too must have at least one parent or guardian who is currently receiving Social Security benefits.

If the child is unmarried.

Medicare eligibility for non-U.S. citizens

Fortunately, even if an individual is not a citizen of the United States it is still possible to receive Medicare if they are eligible to claim because of their current circumstances. The person concerned may still be able to apply for and receive Medicare benefits if they qualify for or are currently receiving Social Security retirement benefits (SSR), Railroad Retirement benefits (RRB), or if the individual is receiving SSDI. If this is the case, the person claiming will qualify for Premium-free Part A. However, with that premium the claimant will owe a premium for Part B insurance. A premium is basically the amount that the individual must pay to the Medicare or another health insurance via a private company for health coverage. Payments to premium plans are usually paid via a monthly fee into the claimants' insurance plan to help cover the Medicare costs.

Medicare eligibility for Part B if the claimant is ineligible for Premium-free Part A

For those who may lack a record of past or recent work history that is currently required to claim and receive Premium-free Part A, Medicare, or they lack the financial resources to pay for hospital insurance because of its monthly payments being too high for their current income. They can still purchase Medicare Part B, which is basic medical insurance without hospital insurance. This form of Medicare payment plan is available as long as the individual can satisfy the following aspects involved with making the claim:

The individual is 65 years old, or older.

The claimant is considered a U.S. citizen or has been residing in the U.S. for five years or more.

Furthermore, if the claimant did not enroll in Part A, Medicare when they first became eligible, and at the point of eligibility a premium needed to be paid to satisfy the claimants Part A plan. The person concerned can only enroll later if they have been offered a 'Special Enrolment Period', or at the time of the General Enrolment Period. However if the person can afford the outlay and is willing to pay the initial Part A premium and therefore wants to be enrolled, they must also take Part B as it is not possible to purchase Part A without Part B Medicare. But if the claimant currently receives Part A Premium-free plan, the individual then has the choice to enroll in Part B if they wish to do so. There are state-specific programs that are available to help those that are on lower incomes and for individuals who have no known assets that may help to cover the costs, and for people who are not eligible for Premium-Free Part A coverage. The 'State Health Insurance Assistance Program', (SHIAP) may be able to help if the claimant resides in New York. The first port of call might be to contact and set up an appointment with the 'Medicare Rights Centre' who will assist in finding and establishing a cost-saving program for the individual making the claim.

Medicare eligibility for Drug Benefit

If the claimant is eligible for Medicare coverage then they are also eligible to claim Medicare drug benefit Part D. But to qualify for this form of health coverage the person must either be currently enrolled in the Medicare Part A or the Part B plan. And unfortunately, Medicare drug coverage is only available via private company plans at this moment in time. Therefore if the individual wants to receive the best beneficial features from the drug benefit coverage and they have Part A and/or Part B, they should automatically enroll in the Part D drug benefit Medicare. This feature will cover the cost of prescription drugs, etc.

Traveling with Medicare

Your Medicare coverage of care when you decide to travel will depend on where you travel and how you actually receive your Medicare benefits. If you are currently in receipt of Original Medicare, then you can travel anywhere in the U.S. This will also include the 50 states, the District of Columbia, the Virgin Islands, American Samoa, Puerto Rico, Guam, and the Northern Marina Islands. And most of the doctor's surgeries and hospitals in these areas will accept your Medicare coverage, on the Original plan.

If you are currently in receipt of the Medicare Advantage plan, then this plan may or may not cover the costs of your care if you are classed as outside of its service area. Some Mcdicare plans may also cover providers that are classed as out-of-the-network areas. But there may be some added costs associated with high cost-sharing – co-payments and co-insurances. The current plan that you are on may also impose certain rules and/or restrictions, like prior authorization. It is best to contact your plan provider to see which rules apply and the cost it entails when you travel within the United States.

If you decide to travel outside of the U.S. where your Medicare plan is not covered for more than six months, then you will automatically be disenrolled from most plans, so that is something to be very cautious about. Albeit, you will have a special enrollment period to let you join a different Medicare plan.

Some Medicare Advantage plans may provide special benefits that will allow you to stay in your current plan if you continuously travel in the United States and all of its territories for up to a maximum of twelve months. You must check the rules and restrictions closely to see if your current plan offers those travel benefits.

Traveling outside the U.S. and Medicare does not usually cover medical care. But the Original Medicare and the Medicare Advantage plans must officially cover the costs of the care that you receive if it includes the following:

Medicare coverage will pay for your medical care if you are on a cruise ship. Only if you get that care if the ship is situated inside the U.S. and Canada.

Medicare coverage will pay for emergency services coverage in Canada if you are traveling via a direct route from the U.S.

In certain situations, Medicare coverage may cover the costs for non-emergency inpatient services in a foreign hospital, and for the ambulance costs if the hospital is closer to the border, e.g. Mexico or Canada, etc.

Medicare Advantage plans may also cover the costs of emergency care when you are abroad in exceptional circumstances. The best thing to do is to contact your care plan provider for more information on this process of costs and coverage in a foreign country.

Medicare coverage is basically broken down into four main parts, which are Medicare Parts A – B – C – D. Finding the right Health, Medicare and/or Life insurance at the lowest price to fit your needs should be the individual's main goal. Each Medicare part will provide its own unique coverage with different benefits and features. And depending on what part which substantially fits the bill for you, the enrollment options will also vary with each particular part. These various Medicare parts may look quite confusing to the uninitiated, but there is no need to worry as you will eventually become an expert in each concept and the processes involved in health insurance once you make the decision to purchase Medicare coverage.

Medicare is a lot like the basic health insurance coverage that you may have already had via an employer or plans you have bought personally in the past. Coverage can cover factors that include visiting your doctor, dental appointments, vision, inpatient and outpatient hospital care, lab tests and prescription drugs, etc. The different parts of Medicare obviously provide different types of health insurance. Before we break down each part it is important to realize that there are enrollment periods. When an individual is nearing the age of 65, they are eligible to enroll in Medicare at three months before their 65th birthday to three months after the date. This is called the Initial Enrollment Period, (IEP). The IEP is the first time that it is possible for you to sign up for Medicare coverage. There is also a General Election Period, (GEP), which allows the person to enroll in Parts A and B. However, there are late penalties that may apply at this Enrollment stage which could increase the premiums on the Medicare coverage that is being purchased. The GEP is available from January 1st to March 31st, and the Medicare coverage will begin on July 1st. Another possible period available to enroll in at the Open Enrollment Period, (OEP). The OEP is available from October 15th to December the 7th. And the Medicare coverage will start covering the individual on January 1st. This period is also known as the Annual Election Period, (AEP). This is the period when individuals can also change their Medicare Advantage and/or their Part D plans. It is also possible at this period to switch from Original Medicare to Medicare Advantage, or vice versa.

As we have already covered, an individual may also be eligible for Medicare at a younger age if they suffer from ESRD or they have a disability that entitles them to make a claim for coverage. When the person applies for Social Security benefits in the U.S. they are automatically enrolled in Medicare Part A. That individual can also choose to enroll in Part B if they would like to receive more coverage for a set premium. These Parts A / B are the Original Medicare plans. With the other parts C / D, they are managed by private insurance companies, enrollment in Part C and D are optional to the individual claimant of Medicare coverage. Medicare Part C is known as Medicare Advantage, which is currently an all-in-one plan that provides both the initial services which are covered by Part A and B Medicare. Part D is basically prescription drug coverage. Searching for and finding the right Medicare coverage depends on what medical services you actually want to be covered for:

Medicare Part A – Hospital Insurance; this coverage will apply to inpatient hospital visits. Coverage of skilled nursing care, home health care, and hospice care.

Medicare Part B – Medical Insurance; will cover doctor visits, outpatient care, lab tests, medical equipment, and ambulance services. Medicare Part B is the only component that initially requires beneficiaries to pay a regular monthly premium payment.

Medicare Part C – Medicare Advantage; which can cover medical insurance, hospital insurance, vision appointments, dental care. and prescription drugs. However, the coverage may not apply to all of the above plans, unless that particular coverage is taken by the individual claimant.

Medicare Part D – Prescription Drugs; this part of the plan will only cover the cost of prescription drugs that the person receives due to an illness.

Before choosing a particular plan, the claimant may need to ask themselves some basic related questions to make sure they are covered for their annual Medicare needs:

Can you afford the plan for out-of-pocket expenses?

Is it possible to keep my current health insurance providers when you swap to Medicare coverage?

Will you need to have a Medicare plan that provides coverage when you travel abroad?

Which hospitals and/or doctors are relevant and are they close enough to visit regularly?

By contacting a licensed insurance agent concerning all the questions that you have, the agent will help you to make the right decision that best suits all of your coverage needs.

Medicare is unlike Social Security as in there are no incentives to defer enrollment past the age of 65 years old. Some social security claimants may elect to receive their benefits before the date of their full retirement age, which is currently at the age of 67, or after. If it is after the age of 67 years old then there may be a penalty towards the claim. If you are an individual who is planning for retirement, you may wish to visit your local social security office and they will provide you with all the information that is needed to ensure the correct claim/s are made concerning what your actual benefit entitlements are. The social security may also help to maximize the benefits that you currently receive.

If for some reason there is a delay in the enrollment process of a Medicare claim the individual might incur an increase on the monthly premiums, especially in the case of Medicare Part B, after enrollment has been completed. To date, senior citizens in the U.S. pay slightly over $100 on a monthly basis for Medicare Part B coverage. But this insurance fee will increase by at least 10% if the enrollment process has encountered a delay of one year. 20% for a two-year delay, etc. Penalties will not be levied on a Part B premium if the person is still in work at the age of 65, and they have cover from their employer's company health insurance plan. The same non-levies are applied if the beneficiary is covered under their spouse's employer's health insurance. However, with that, the person will be subject to the 'special enrollment period'. As a claimant, you may find that paying the fee for a monthly premium for a Medicare Part B plan is worth the outlay, due to the amount you will save in out-of-pocket expenses. If your current employer's health insurance group plan is your main healthcare coverage, and you wish to take more time before enrollment in the Medicare initiative of Part B, then you should definitely enroll in Medicare Part A once you reach the age of 65 years old because there will be no fee for a premium, even though the extra hospital coverage is available to you.

If you are the claimant and you are over the age of 65, and not currently working but you still retain a health insurance policy via your former employer, then it is wise to still enroll in a Medicare plan. Because in the case of a retiree plan, that would be your secondary health insurance plan, but you will still have the need for Medicare coverage to help you pay for future health care expenses that may occur in your later years. Senior citizens who are already claiming social security benefits will automatically be enrolled in Medicare coverage. The cards that are associated with the insurance plan will be sent to you in the mail about three months before your 65th birthday arrives. If you, the claimant are not in receipt of social security benefits, you should quickly apply for Medicare at the three months before the date to ensure that you do not receive any additional penalties because of lack any discrepancies like lack of correspondence from the Social Security Administration. It may be best to keep up to date with any plan you think you may be entitled too by regularly visiting your social security office or by going online at regular intervals before your 65th birthday.

If you are lucky enough to be currently in the earning bracket of more than $90.000 in annual income, then, unfortunately, you will definitely be subject to a surcharge in your Medicare coverage no matter which plan/s you choose to enroll on. For joint claimants, the surcharge cap is currently at an estimated $185.000 in annual income between you both. These surcharges can certainly add up, and they will not only be present in a Medicare Part B claim, but also to the Medicare Part C plan. And unfortunately, it will also be involved in a basic prescription drug benefit which entails the Part D plan of Medicare coverage. These substantial surcharges can get quite expensive as it is averaged at about $500 just for the Part B Medicare health insurance coverage. Quite costly in my opinion, and I am sure that you would agree.

If you are a senior who is currently below the higher wage bracket, or you are on quite a low income, you may find that the average plan can cost around $110 on a monthly basis for the premium Medicare plans, which could be well above your budget. If so, you might be able to apply and qualify for the Medicare Savings Program, (MSP). The program is basically a system that is financially supported by the U.S. state to provide much-needed help for seniors with low income, and who wish to claim Medicare coverage. Although Medicaid is available too, I would advise you that I think Medicare is the best option for low-income seniors in need of state aid. And it is also possible for disabled individuals to receive help from the state via these initiatives. State-funded programs will include:

Qualified disabled and working individuals program

Qualified individual program

Qualified Medicare Beneficiary program

Specified low-income Medicare Beneficiary program

If after the enrollment period in Medicare Part A / B is complete, there may be no need for you to enroll in a Part D plan unless that is what you actually want to do.

In the case of the Medicare Part C plan, which is officially known as Medicare Advantage. This coverage currently allows private insurance companies to basically offer health coverage via a contract with Medicare and other healthcare insurers. Private corporations can provide plans that are specialized to cater to your current insurance needs. These privately-owned health insurers that offer the Medicare Advantage plan have an incentive to make you feel comfortable with the plan you choose, and they will help you to get the best deal on the market when you enroll, claim and receive coverage from their company insurance policy. Therefore, you may get a great deal of discount for Plan C Medicare if you can choose the right company for you, and your current income.

The Initial Enrollment Period (IEP) for Medicare coverage is available, but if for some reason you may have missed that time-period, then it is still possible to enroll in the General Enrollment Period, (GEP) at any given year from January 1st, all the way through to March 31st, without surcharges and/or potential premium fees interrupting your benefits.

The Hospital has several responsibilities, one being good stewards of hospital resources. The other is being a good steward of the Pt's resources. Meaning that in the United States there are 5,534 hospitals, 2,849 hospitals are not for profit, 1,035 are for profit. But, they all have to monitor cost in one-way shape or form. We also have to be careful of your Medicare Days for hospital and skilled nursing facilities.

For the Hospital, you have one hundred hospital days per episode. When you are discharged from the hospital you will have to be out of the hospital for sixty days. Then your hospital days will reload. Hospitals have run into the unique situation that a patient has run out of hospital days due to severe illness. At that point, the patient will get a bill from the hospital. The Hospitals, Physicians and Case Managers have done everything in their power to work with the Pt and family to come up with a better solution for the Pt.

When you have to visit hospital due to an illness, and they decide to keep you in that hospital to treat you, then you will be assigned with a file tag with either an observation status or an inpatient status. To be assigned as observation status it is likely that you are basically not really sick enough to be considered inpatient status, or the illness does not require specialist care, therefore there is no need to keep you in the hospital to monitor the illness. It may even be that your doctor does not know exactly what the sickness is, so they wish to simply observe you, and see if your illness becomes any worse. To be assigned as an inpatient in the hospital, then it is highly likely that you may be suffering from an illness, or you may have had a severe accident that requires skilled health care treatment, and it may need regular medical attention on the hospital wing.

Observation patients are basically a type of outpatient, most hospitals in the United States will have a specialist patient observation area or a medical wing for their observation patients to visit regularly to help monitor their progress. However, many hospitals may put the observation patients in the same area as the inpatients, this can generally cause some confusion between the patients because one might think that they are now an observation patient when they are really an inpatient, and visa versa. This confusion is enhanced due to the fact that an observation patient can actually be in the hospital for several days, but they are still not considered as an inpatient. Albeit. Observation is intended for very short stays, however, it is not always like that. The only way to know for sure if you are considered as observation status or as inpatient status is if you ask the medical team who are dealing with your illness. It can be quite confusing at the best of times, because hospitals and even your local doctor cannot simply assign you to one status or another without doing their due diligence and sticking to the medical guidelines concerning whatever it is the illness is that you are currently suffering from and whether it warrants an observation, or inpatient status.

Both statuses have different criteria. It is about the severity of the illness, and whether or not you are sick enough to need specialist inpatient care with longer-term hospital admission. It can also relate to the intensity of the illness in question and the amount of service needed from the medical team to control the illness and to help you to make a full recovery. A hospital stay will let the team evaluate and utilize the illness. The nurse in charge of your care will compare your doctor's findings, look into your current diagnosis, and determine if it is correct. The nurse may take more tests and do new studies searching for results concerning your sickness and how to overcome as soon as possible. Only after all tests are completed, reviewed, and the illness is determined, will you, the patient be either assigned as an observation patient or an inpatient of the hospital.

If your illness is bad enough to warrant a stay in hospital as an inpatient, but your Medicare coverage has determined that you should have been assigned as an observation patient instead of the inpatient status, then this can have a detrimental effect on your coverage. Because Medicare may then refuse to pay for the entire stay in the hospital when you were considered as an inpatient. Unfortunately, if that is the case then you may be out of pocket, and you might not discover that you are now in healthcare debt until the hospital submits the claim for expenses to your Medicare insurance coverage provider. Which will effectively be denied by Medicare after they receive the claim. This can happen months after your hospitalization period. So, with that information at hand, it would always be wiser to ask as soon as possible whether you are an observation patient or an inpatient, and if your current status is the correct one for your illness.

Observation patients are like outpatients so the medical bills are covered by the Medicare Part B plan. This kind of observation coverage can have higher coinsurance rates than the inpatient status Medicare coverage. This is true if your Part B plan has the coinsurance with the no out-of-pocket cap included in the coverage. Or, unless you are currently on the Medicare Advantage plan - Part C. If that is the case, you may have to pay a larger amount of the medical bill for the observation status and the service it provides, than you would have paid for a hospital inpatient service with a longer-term stay. A result like that can certainly be very frustrating, but the best way to combat any confusion in status and/or if your hospital status meets your Medicare coverage and your current budget is to make sure that you have been assigned the correct status for the illness you are suffering from.

It is more advantageous to be assigned as an inpatient if you are receiving Medicare coverage and if you may need some time in a nursing facility after the hospitalization. But if that is not the case, and your illness is likely to be short-term, then it may be best to fight for observation status rather than inpatient status to help make sure that all of your medical costs can be covered by your current Medicare plan.

You may also feel that you have to fight for the Inpatient status. Again, the status is going to be assigned by the admitting physician. It will also be checked by the Case Manager on the floor. If the Hospitalist or Case Manager intentionally place you in a status that you do not qualify for. It could be considered Medicare Fraud, which would be five years in jail and $250,000. The offender would also lose their license.

If you are not the patient, and it is your mom or dad who has to be admitted into the hospital, then a determination will be made by the medical team to decide whether their stay is assigned the observational status or the inpatient status. The best thing for you to do is to be present at that illness determination appointment to help your parent to understand the process and the results that they receive from the hospital staff. Your mom or dad may not fully understand the technicalities of what the medical team is stating and what it may mean/cost to their Medicare plan coverage. If you are there to help guide them through the entire process, then your parent will also feel more at ease in the hospital environment with you by their side. If the result of their illness means that they have been assigned as an observation patient, then you will need to inform your mom or dad that their Medicare plan may not cover their current status as Medicare does not really consider observation status as an admission and therefore they do not fully cover the costs as the coverage would if they were admitted as an inpatient. If that is the case, your parent may be charged for their illness determination visit. They may even be asked to pay in cash at the appointment, which can be quite a shock if you are not aware of that Medicare concept. Furthermore, the cash outlay for an observation patient is far more than the initial cost for an inpatient, and the insurance reimbursements may not pay out. If they do, it will only be a small percentage of the actual cost of the observational visit. That is because all insurance companies including Medicare coverage currently negotiate much lower rates to the hospitals than the patients actually pay for their Medicare coverage. It is a fact that Medicare does not fully reimburse hospitals for patient costs, especially when they are readmitted within 30 days of leaving the hospital, and/or after their first determination visit to provide the observation or inpatient status. And this is why hospital mainly put patients on observational status so they can avoid the potential of being penalized from the insurance company if the patient returns to the hospital after they were given an inpatient status by the medical team.

For information concerning your mom or dad's Medicare coverage, and whether it will cover the costs of care without them being hit by a substantial sum after the initial hospital visit/stay, you should pay particular attention to these associated factors:

The out-of-pocket costs can become much higher for the patient if they are on Medicare, and they are not admitted into the hospital. This is likely if the Medicare Plan B is the only coverage in use for the patient. To receive most of the cost from their coverage, your mom or dad would have to be formally admitted into the hospital for a stay of at least two days. If they are, and it is only under the observation status then this designation can actually compromise the care your parent receives because they have not formally been admitted into the hospital, therefore your mom or dad is not fully covered by Medicare as they are not fully part of the process of receiving the medical care for patients that is needed to cover the health costs.

Medicare coverage can also be compromised if the hospital stay is slightly more than two days, and they are only considered as under observation because the insurance reimbursements can become so low once the patient receives a certain amount of care. It is wise to note this fact, as many patients can be sent home before they have fully recovered from their illness in the hope of recovering at home in your care, or in a healthcare facility.

If it is highly likely that your mom or dad is a patient receiving Medicare coverage, and he/she must be admitted into a local nursing home/healthcare facility, then your parent/s are required to be hospitalized as an inpatient for a certain amount of time prior to the healthcare facility admission, if they wish for the Medicare coverage to full pay for their stay in a nursing home. But if you think it best for your parent/s to be admitted into a nursing home and they have only been given the observational status, then sadly there will be no healthcare reimbursements paid by the Medicare plan to the facility taking care of the patient. These costs can actually to hundreds of thousands of dollars, or even more. So, the best option here would be to fight for your parent/s status to be raised from observation to inpatient status. Your mom or dad must be formally admitted and hospitalized for at least three days in this circumstance for them to receive the cost of care on their Medicare plan's insurance policy.

Several years ago, there used to be a clear distinction between the observation and inpatient status. the patient who was admitted into the hospital was classified as an inpatient, and the patient who was treated in hospital but sent home to fully recover was classified as an outpatient under the observation service. The observation status was originally introduced by the Center of Medicare and Medicaid services. For the patients who were Medicare beneficiaries, and those who were treated in the emergency room at the hospital were considered observation patients even if they had to have more than 24 hours of hospital care. But now there is a sort of in-between status that is addressed to two issues:

The cost of care – Medicare recently lowered its payment to hospitals for the shorter hospital stays, i.e. 24+ hours.
The appropriateness of care – observation status had given doctors and nurses more time to actually figure out whether the patient needs to be admitted into the hospital for a longer period of time for ongoing care and treatment. Or, if the patient could stay on observation status and sent home after discharge to fully recover.

With that new in-between status, it did not take long before the hospital administrators discovered ways to use the in-between observation status to their advantage. They quickly realized that by placing a patient in observation instead of in the inpatient category, the hospital could then avoid the financial penalty levied for Medicare coverage patients who for some reason had to return for e re-admission within the penalized 30 days term. And Medicare also denies any payment to hospitals for the patient who they think has been classified in the wrong category and discharged after a 48-hour period in hospital. These both create incentives for hospitals to place the patient in the observation status. even with those patients who have stayed in the hospital for longer than 48 hours.

Cost of observation and inpatient care:

As the costs of inpatient care are rapidly growing on a yearly basis, Medicare coverage beneficiaries are likely to revisit observation care instead of being hospitalized with inpatient status. this is a current trend that potential has unforeseen financial implications for the people who receive Medicare coverage because observation care, although it is classed as typically hospital-based care by most Medicare claimants, it is actually classified as an outpatient care service. Therefore the claimants of Medicare who are readmitted into hospital actually pay the inpatient deductible every benefit period.

Claimants who have multiple care visits and under the observation status are subject to the coinsurance fee at every stay and these fees can substantially add up to a high cumulative cost annually. On average, the beneficiaries of Medicare coverage who have multiple observation stays in hospital, and at a 60 period, can have a cumulative cost liability of $947.40, and more than %26 of beneficiaries had a financial liability that exceeded the inpatient deductibles. And Medicare beneficiaries with multiple stays in hospital over a 60-day period have a higher cumulative cost liability than they would have had if they were actually claiming the Medicare Part A plan.

Albeit, observation care is normally delivered to the patient as an outpatient service which is covered by Part B Medicare rather than the Part A plan for inpatient care. More than half of the hospitals in the United States treat the observation status as an administrative classification above all else. This care can also be delivered on the same wings as the inpatient service. Therefore, the patients are often unaware of their status, as we have already discussed in an early chapter. But this kind of misconception can cause the patient a lot of frustration, and it can also have financial implications when the patient receives their hospital bill. The implications have the potential to cause an impact to the Medicare's liability via four different mechanisms.

Instead of the expected fixed cost for admission at the inpatient status, which is classed as a fixed deductible for the hospital stay, the patient will have to pay a high percentage of each service they receive while in the hospital's care, and for the treatment, they are issued. Therefore the Medicare patient who may have had long observation stays, or who receives an expensive course of treatment may have to pay a very high financial liability to cover the costs as Medicare will not pay out.

2. Medicare does not cover the exact same services whilst the patient is in hospital, e.g. observation care is different from inpatient care. Consider self-administered medications, these are not covered for Medicare beneficiaries who are at the observation status during their hospitalization. The cost of services is considerably cheaper at for the patient who has been officially admitted into the hospital. Self-administered medications are covered by Medicare at inpatient status.

3. There are certain beneficial features that some Medicare claimants are not eligible to receive unless they have been officially admitted into the hospital for several days. For the patient to receive

Medicare cover for nursing facilities after their stay in the hospital. They must have been hospitalized for three or more days.

4. Medicare coverage beneficiaries who have to revisit hospital will have greater cumulative costs as covered above. Although some Medicare coverage will protect you from high culminative costs under the observation status vs the inpatient status, this is known as the benefit period. A benefit period will begin on the day that the patient is admitted into a hospital or admitted into a nursing home after hospitalization. This benefit period will then end after a 60-day stay. But the patient is likely to pay the inpatient deductible fee once during their benefit period. This fee is only paid once, even if the patient has multiple readmissions during that time.

If a Medicare beneficiary is considered as an outpatient/observation status and is currently in receipt of Medicare Part B, then they are covered by their insurance plan to receive that care without any cost. Whilst if the beneficiary is in receipt of Part A, the beneficiary will be covered for all costs under the inpatient status. Therefore, if the beneficiary is currently receiving Medicare Part A but is not in receipt of the Part B plan, then that person will have to pay the full costs of their hospitalization whilst they are still only classified at the observational status.

Being in the observation status can have a significant impact on your hospital bill and it is associated with an increase in out-of-pocket expenses. The observation status is an outpatient status, and certain insurance companies handle the observation status very differently from the inpatient status. Medicare insurance will cover some cost of the observation status in their Part B coverage if the status is the correct one issued by the hospital. The inpatient status is covered in full by Medicare Part A coverage. This is paid in full after the patient has paid a single deductible fee.

With each outpatient/observation hospital service, they all have separate co-payments, these co-payments can really add up and they can exceed the deductible for inpatient care status. the Medicare patient who is in the observation status is liable for paying 20% of the cost of care after they have paid the deductible. Whilst inpatients and the medications that they are provided with during their hospitalization are all covered under the Medicare Part A plan, they are not covered for those patients who are on observation even if they have Part A and Part B Medicare. Patients without Medicare Part D prescription drug coverage, they will find themselves having to pay the out-of-pocket fees for their medications. And the patient who currently has private health insurance will have to face much higher bills than those on Medicare for observation status care. The system is a bit wayward, but the most important thing to remember is that the days you spend on the observation status do not count towards the required three-day minimum hospital stay/nursing home care for Medicare coverage to pay the medical bills.

No matter what status you are placed in at the hospital, the treatment will still be the same. Hospitals are there to treat the patient with the best care possible and without discrimination. Whether it is you, your mom, or your dad is in the hospital's care, and you/they are either in observation or as an inpatient of the hospital, the doctors and nurses have a duty of care, and a duty to make your stay in hospital as comfortable as possible. You, the patient, will receive first class care from well-trained professionals who are people that really do care about your health and well-being. hospital staff deserves all the credit that they receive because the job they do each day is a job that deserves respect. You or your parents will be in the best possible hands, and they will help you to a full recovery as quickly as they can.

After hospital care, many seniors are unable to return home because they need further health care to help them recover from their illness. A stay in a nursing home may be required to ensure the health and safety of your parent/s. This rehabilitation period may be necessary for your mom or dad until their medical condition stabilizes. If so, for Medicare to cover these costs, the patient/s must have spent at least the three-day term in the hospital before they go to nursing care. And that hospital stay must have been under the inpatient status. Many Medicare enrollees that are in receipt of the benefits are still receiving large medical bills for their time in a nursing home facility. That is because these enrollees have not met the inpatient criteria to ensure the full cost of care is covered by their Medicare plans. So, that is definitely something to keep in mind before admitting your mom or dad into a nursing home facility. To make matters more complicated, your parent/s may be in the observation status and actually think that they are in the inpatient status due to its confusion between patients. The admission status is not often discussed by doctors and/or nurses with the patient, therefore, it is a matter that I suggest you make completely sure of the correct category for your parent/s with the medical staff in the hospital. As we have already discussed, some hospitals do not have designated areas and they may put the observation patients in the same area as the patients with inpatient status. Albeit, Medicare has tried to address this confusion by creating and enacting a law that now requires notification to the patient who is currently receiving care in the observation status category, and the hospital staff are now supposed to talk to the patient about the implications to the Medicare coverage plan, and the observation status fees. But that may not be the case when you visit the hospital, because it is a new law that may take some time for medical staff to get used to. And this law has no such rules for the patient who receives health insurance from a private company.

The very best way for you or your parent/s to avoid being blindsided by this Medicare law is to make sure that you are well informed. Talk to the staff as soon as you visit the hospital, and when you are admitted. You will be admitted under the observation or inpatient status, so speak to staff and find out exactly which category you are in to guarantee Medicare coverage will cover the costs for your stay in the hospital and in a nursing home facility. Also, your medical status can change form time to time, so be aware of that fact too. The status can change due to the fact that your illness has become worse or the fact that you are getting better and your health is currently improving by the quality care that you have received. Whilst there is nothing you can actually do to modify your current status upon admission, you can still do a lot by making sure that you have the correct information as it will allow you to prepare for the financial implications, and it will help you to avoid being completely by surprise if you receive a large medical bill. The best bet would be to contact your insurance company for a brief explanation of your benefit entitlements whilst you are in either the observation or inpatient category. The Medicare coverage should inform you of the out-of-pocket costs by giving you an estimate of the likely charges for your care under both statuses.

The observation service is basically a short-term outpatient service, which is received when a patient is in the hospital, and the patient is being monitored to determine whether or not that patient should be admitted as in inpatient. It is very important to realize that you are receiving observation care and you are not considered an inpatient for Medicare coverage reasons. And even if you are admitted into the hospital for an overnight stay, that still does not mean that you are considered at the inpatient status. Keeping fully informed is the best way to know what status you are at whilst hospitalized. The hospital staff should keep you up to date with your status. There is now a notice that should be issued to patients who receive Medicare coverage. That notice is called the Medicare Outpatient Observation Notice (MOON). The MOON notifies you, as a patient of the hospital, that you are currently on observation, and the notice will notify why you are only considered as an outpatient and not classified in the inpatient status. The medical staff who are in charge of your hospital care should notify you during your hospitalization period. And the fact that the observation service will often involve an overnight stay in the hospital, and that you may still not be considered as an inpatient. The importance of staying up to date with your progression in hospital, i.e. your current status, will keep you informed about the financial implications concerning your Medicare coverage, and if it actually covers the costs of the care you receive.

Medicare Part A will cover all the cost of the care that you receive whilst in the hospital and you are considered an inpatient.
Medicare Part B will cover the costs of the that you receive in whilst in the hospital and you are considered as an outpatient / at the observation status.
You may pay more when Medicare Part B is your only cover for your hospital care.
It is possible to have multiple co-payments. Each individual co-payments must be lower than the Medicare Part A deductible, which is currently at $1.340 in 2018. The total co-pay costs may actually be higher than the Part A deductible, so do be aware of that fact.
Medicare Part B does not cover the costs of the medication that you routinely take. You will need to be covered with the Medicare Part D plan for prescription drug coverage. You may pay more for the drugs at the hospital's pharmacy if you cannot provide proof of your Medicare Part D coverage.
Medicare will not cover the cost of skilled nursing facility care. You must be considered as a hospital inpatient for at least three days

before any cost is covered by Medicare coverage. This basically means that if you have been considered at the observation status whilst you were hospitalized, and then the hospital suggests a stay in a nursing home for you to recover with extra care, then you may receive a very large unexpected bill for that care as Medicare will not pay the costs. Always maintain awareness of your hospital status because you will be liable for the out-of-pocket costs if you have failed to realize that you were on observation and not an actual inpatient during your hospital stay.

If you think that it may be time for you the patient, or for your mom or dad who receives Medicare coverage to set up a power of attorney in your name to make sure that everything concerning the financial aspects of the process is under your control, then you should formally be known as the care provider for the Medicare beneficiary, i.e. your parent/s. many people do not realize that they must be registered as the care and the power of attorney for them to make healthcare-related decisions on behalf of the patient. You as the child to your parent will not be able to enroll in Medicare on your parent's behalf, alongside the fact that you will not be able to appeal on their behalf for Medicare coverage after a hospital visit or a long-term care home stay. Unless you are officially the power of attorney and you, therefore, have the legal power to do so. As the Power of Attorney (POA), you will be required to provide POA proof even if the person in your care is your parent or any other family member, including your spouse, etc. For you to be able to make any healthcare decision for your loved ones, you must be appointed as a legal representative, e.g. their Power of Attorney.

Becoming your mom or dad's POA will give you the power make important healthcare decisions that will be of great benefit to your parent's condition and the current medical care that they receive. Because when you are officially known as your parents' POA you will receive a legal document that will inform the Department of

Health and Human Services that it is you who has the right to represent your parent, and you may even be considered as your parent's legal guardian. Obviously, this will benefit your mom or dad because you will fight for the best care possible to help them overcome the illness they suffer, and you will make sure that all of your parent's financial issues are dealt with accordingly.

Your parent/s may not be capable of dealing with these important factors for themselves, especially if their illness is serious enough to warrant extra care like a nursing home admission. So, becoming your mom or dad's POA can be the best thing to do to enable that you have full control, and you have it legally. If you are considering becoming your parents' power of attorney, then you should be aware that there are several different types of POA documentation which may limit your legal authority. Some only give you the right to manage your parents' finances whilst some only provide the right for healthcare decision-making.

To become POA you will need to make an appointment with a licensed attorney in your local area to discuss the best options. The attorney will provide all the information that you need about it and can quickly give you the POA documentation to fill out and apply for the appropriate POA legality on your behalf. Once that you have filled out all the documentation that is needed by the state, then you should keep them safe. You could even leave a copy with your attorney in case one copy is lost due to unforeseen circumstances. You will need to produce this documentation on certain occasions, like for Medicare coverage and other health insurance, or nursing home care, and financial matters concerning your parent/s.

For Medicare plan representation, you will also need to fill out an Appointment of Representative form. This will authorize you to legally represent your parent/s in Medicare claims, payments, and other important Medicare decisions.

There are different rule and limitations concerning the POA, but you will be informed by your attorney which is the best action for you to take regarding your parent's care. The rules and limitations can differ from state to state in the U.S. but it is possible for you to customize the limits that you have on your parent/s behalf. Generally, a POA documentation agreement will provide you with the following abilities:

Use your parents' money to pay their bills

File your parents' taxes

Operate your parents' businesses

Collect their social security benefits

Manage your parents' investments

Buy, sell, and fully manage the property on your parents' behalf

Conduct banking transactions on their behalf

Manage your parents' retirement benefits and related accounts

Hire professional help to represent them in any matter of legal concern

Give donations to charity in your parents' name

Manage all funds concerning your parents Medicare, and other coverage/treatments

Choosing their health care options and changing health insurance plans

Appealing against any Medicare denial issues

Power of Attorney documentation is valid until either you, your parents, or the state revoke it, which is highly unlikely unless there are fraudulent concerns.

If your parent/s becomes completely incapacitated due to illness, injury or they sadly become deceased unexpectedly, you must be aware that there is the option of creating a durable POA document to guarantee that you have all the responsibilities that are needed to assure the appropriate care is given, and that you have full control over your parents finances after incapacitation or death.

Financial POA:

Becoming your parent/s financial power of attorney will give you the legal right and responsibility to be in control and to take care of their finances during their health care and after their death. As a property and financial POA, you can make decisions on behalf of the person/parent. You can be in control of all the important decisions, and applications that need to be made to ensure the safety of the person's financial well-being. The decisions/applications in your control as financial POA can include:

The person's funds, taxes, and bills.

Their property and investments.

Pensions and Social Security benefits.

Banks and building society account control

You can basically take full control of the individual's money and use those funds to pay their bills, look after their home, pay for healthcare, and purchase day to day products for the person, e.g. food, clothes, etc. As the legal financial POA, you can discuss important decisions that will affect the individual's living arrangements, healthcare factors, and daily routine with their current health and welfare attorney, if the person in care has one. When you become the person's / parent/s POA, you must keep their finances completely separate from your own. Unless you have a legal joint account, or you own your own home together.

Once you have registered as the lasting power of attorney, (LPA), you will then be able to take control of the financial aspects after you have shown the bank/building society a copy of the legally binding document. You will also need to give proof of your name, address, and the individual's name and address who is under your financial care, alongside their bank account details, the bank may ask for more proof concerning your POA liability, but the documentation that you produce should be enough for the bank to issue an account that gives you the right to use the individual's funds if it is legit, and therefore state approved.

Living Will:

The term 'Living Will' refers to the legal documentation that provides the person with the capability to state their wishes for their end-of-life medical care. The living will also be known as the 'Health Care Directive', and/or the 'Advanced Directive'.

The living will is not like an ordinary will that people use to leave an inheritance to their loved ones, it is a directive to medical physicians, and the document basically lets people state their personal wishes in case they become incapacitated and they are unable to communicate their medical decisions. This documentation has no power after the death of the person. If it is your parents in hospital and they are suffering from a potentially life-threatening illness, then making a living will be a very valuable factor to make sure that your parents' wishes are fully understood and followed to their every word. The living will also give invaluable advice and guidance about your parents' estate, and guidance for family members, and the healthcare professionals that are providing your parents care. It is a will that expresses those end-of-life wishes, without a living will document of expression, family members and medical professionals are basically left to guess what the person would prefer in terms of their medical treatment. This can cause friction between family members which can occasionally end up in a court battle.

The requirements for a living will vary from state to state, but the best thing to do is hire a professional lawyer to inform you about the full process and to help you, and/or your parents prepare the living will. However, it is possible to create a living will on your own accord. With the correct software application, and one that accounts for your state's laws, it is quite easy to make a living will without the need for the large legal fees that a lawyer may charge for this service. You can create a legally binding living will without paying those high fees by using a reputable estate planning software. Something like WillMaker Plus will suffice. And in addition to making a living will, you could also create a set of estate planning documents. This documentation includes legalities like a will, the power of attorney, their living trust, etc.

Many states in the U.S. have certain forms that are for advance directives. These forms will allow the person to state their full wishes in as much detail as they want to provide to their family members, or maybe only to the health professionals who are caring for them. And for the living will to be valid, it must meet the state requirements regarding the notarization, and witnesses of the documentation. A living will can be revoked at any time. It can also take effect immediately after creation, and as soon as the document is signed by all concerned. Or, it may only take effect when the person can no longer communicate their wishes due to severe illness, etc.

The living will is often used with the document that is called a durable power of attorney, (DPOA). This document is aimed at the POA for the person's healthcare. The DPOA can appoint someone to carry out the person's wishes, just like the living will. In fact, the two documents are usually combined together to give full authority to the POA to carry out the individual who is considered at the end-of-life treatment stage in their care. The person who is named on the documentation is called the 'agent', or the 'healthcare proxy'.

The full authority that is granted by the living will ends when the individual sadly becomes deceased.

Getting extra help in times of need can make life much easier for all concerned. Private duty nursing is the care of clients by nurses who may be currently licensed as registered nurses, (RNs), or licensed practical nurses, (LPNs / LVNs). Most of these nurses who provide the private duty care will often work on a one-to-one basis with the patient. And the care may be provided in the patient's home or in another facility like a nursing home or other healthcare institution. The private duty care may be paid via a private company that the person receives their private health insurance from. Or, by a managed healthcare organization like that of Medicare, and Medicaid. Many of the private duty nurses are actually self-employed individuals who work for private contractors in the home healthcare profession. But there are also the governmental nurses who offer home nursing care and care for patients in the many homes that the government currently provide for those in need.

The private duty care field is a home care service that is provided to the elderly, or to those with certain disabilities who are in need of professional assistance with their everyday activities. The private duty nurse will visit the patient's home and help them with things such as meal preparation, personal grooming, and the patient's hygiene, and housekeeping issues. The duty nurse will also provide companionship to those who are in need of a friend in what can be very difficult times during their elderly life, and/or because of their current illness. A private duty nurse may also offer transport to and from healthcare appointments, or to certain places that the patient wants to visit. This kind of home help can really make the difference to the patient lifestyle. And in some cases, the nurse will provide physical, and mental health therapy services to the client. However, that will depend on the private agencies home care objectives and the service that they offer to that particular patient.

Choosing a private duty care agency/nurse for your loved one is a good option that will help to ensure their personal safety, and their comfort whilst they are still living in their own home. The nurse in charge of the private care will work with you to assess your current need, and/or the needs of your parent/s, and the family in general. The nurse will then try to satisfy all the goals that have been set to provide the very best medical, physical, and emotional care possible to the patient. The nurse in charge of care will be well trained and very experienced, and they would have been subjected to a criminal background check in the past for safety reasons, etc.

In order to access the needs of your loved ones, you will need to discuss every option that is available to help the private duty nurse make the best possible arrangements for their care plan. A care plan will be set by the nurse to assist the patient with the following objectives in mind:

To assist the individual with maintaining proper personal hygiene, consisting of bathing, grooming, laundry services, cooking, and other similar tasks.

Reminding the patient to take all of their prescribed medication.

Provide transport to certain events such as medical appointments, and personal visits, i.e. family visits, etc.

Assist with shopping for groceries, and other messages.

Assisting in housekeeping and maintenance issues.

Provide professional and friendly companionship.

If the time has arrived for you, or your parent/s to consider private duty home care nursing services, then you should research more about how in-home-care can truly benefit the person's life. It is a great service that many people with private duty care experiences speak very highly of. This is because of many individuals whether they are elderly and/or they are disabled, etc, they enjoy living in their own home and prefer it to live in a nursing facility. Private duty care allows the patient to do that whilst they are also receiving the help from a healthcare professional.

Nursing Home Facilities:

Only recently, Medicare has issued several national coverage determinations that provide its different insurance coverage for the services and the procedures of a complex nature, with the stipulation that all facilities under the Medicare wing provide a service that meets the current Medicare criteria. This criteria requires that the nursing home facility meets the minimum standards to ensure the safety of Medicare beneficiaries who are in nursing homes in order to be considered as a care provider with the ability to perform professional care procedures. And being a certified care provider that is considered as a Medicare-approved facility, it is required by law for the care home to be capable of performing the following care procedures to ensure all residents receive the appropriate care:

Managing health and safety
Providing medication
Physical Therapy
Occupational Therapy
Memory Care
Administer care plans

As you can see by the above procedures, these nursing home facilities must be able to fully care for their residents, including the care of performing important procedures. So, it is very likely that you, the patient, or your parent/s will be in the best possible care if you choose a Medicare-approved facility to administer the care.

If it is time to start considering a potential care facility, then you will have to have an assessment before this service becomes available to the patient. The purpose of this medical assessment is to evaluate and determine what resources are needed to administer the proper care for the patient whilst he/she is a resident of the nursing home facility. This valuation will include day-to-day care and care in emergency situations. The assessment will constantly be reviewed and updated when necessary. Using this competency-based approach is to enable the nursing staff to assure that each resident is receiving the individual care that allows the patient to maintain their physical, mental and psychological well-being whilst they are in the facility.

A nursing home facility is for people who do not need to be in hospital but they cannot be cared for at home due to certain matters concerning their health and safety. Most of these nursing home facilities have nursing aides and highly skilled nurses on hand 24 hours a day to care for the residents. The care home staff will provide full medical care including speech, physical, psychological, and occupational therapy to their patients. Some of these nursing home facilities are actually set-up like a hospital while others try to make it more like a home from home experience. They initially try to have a neighborhood feel to their facility to make the residents feel comfortable while they are in their care. The staff in a nursing home facility may be encouraged to develop relationships with their residents to make them feel loved and appreciated. Most care homes provide special units for patients who may suffer from serious memory loss problems like Alzheimer's disease, etc. Some care facilities will even let couples/partners live together in the residence. These home are not only considered for the elderly, but they are also for anyone who is in need of 24-hour help and care.

Before choosing a nursing home facility for yourself or your parent/s you should make sure that the facility is the right one for you and your family, and that the facility will provide you or your parent/s with the best possible care. Nursing homes are a valuable option when the amount of medical care and attention the patient needs cannot be provided within the comfort of their own home because of certain issues that may include, frequent incontinence, the inability to sleep through the night, dangerous wanderings, and mental instability. If this is the case and it is your parent/s who need specialist care and attention from professional medical staff, and in a nursing facility, then choosing the right home is paramount to ensure that your parent/s are well looked after, and that they receive professional help that you, yourself cannot provide. But at the same time, you must include your mom or dad into the equation of choosing the most suitable care facility to fit their current needs. If your parent/s is still mentally alert, then he or she must be involved in the process of finding and securing a nursing home that they themselves are happy with. Your parents should have a part and have their say about every single step of the way in their future care predicament. Because moving out of one/s own home and into a care facility is a massive step to take, and it is a considerable change to your parent/s life. Furthermore adjusting to such a move may take time to become completely comfortable with. Both you and your parent/s will need time and patience during this adjustment in care period. Even up to the first month in a nursing home can be quite a struggle for you and your parent/s. This time should be like a trial period for you all to adjust and get used to the new situation and the change in circumstances that a major move like that entails. You should regularly visit your parent/s and try your very best to make them feel at ease. I am sure that you would do anything to make your parent/s feel loved and appreciated in this their time of need, and just being there for them can make such the difference. You can play an important role in assuring that your parent/s receive the quality care that they so deserve. You may want to be as involved as you possibly can in the progression of your parents care whilst in the care facility, you can do that by visiting them often, and speaking to staff on a regular basis, and by participating in care meetings and care planning initiatives. You may even wish to be involved in certain outings that the care home offers to its residents to give your parent/s a better chance of association within the facility.

Finding suitable alternative living arrangements for people who are suffering at home is becoming more difficult as it is a very complex issue for some since there are numerous community resources that provide many different levels of care. Therefore you should research all of your options before deciding which option is best for your parent/s. These resources may vary from community to community and state to state. But with persistence, you will discover the best alternative living arrangements for your parent/s current needs. Also, you should research different funding options/sources for the different types of care facilities. Medicare will cover the costs if your parent/s have spent more than three days in the hospital and the medical staff has decided that the best available option to progress with your parents care is to find a suitable care facility like a nursing home. But it cannot hurt to try to find other options if you or your parent/s do not agree. Or they cannot accept their local nursing home as a suitable living place. Nursing homes are residential care facilities that can certainly differ in many features, and they can provide a wide range of different services. Finding the best one for your parent/s is extremely important.

Both federal and state regulations will require that a doctor or a nurse in charge of your parents care will be capable of routinely visiting your parent/s in the nursing home and assessing them on regular occasions concerning their care and their health status. And all nursing home staff will always be fully trained to cope with any possibility with your parents and with their needs on a 24-hour basis so you can be certain that your parent/s are in the best possible hands.

There are several different types of nursing home care that you might want to consider depending on your parent/s desires and their particular needs. Two of them at your disposal and that is currently the most popular are:

Skilled nursing care – provides 24-hour service by licensed nurses and/or rehabilitation services. These facilities will provide full medical care for both the short-term and the long-term stays in the nursing home. The short-term stay may be straight after hospitalization which could take up to four-six weeks of rehabilitation in the care home facility. And the long-term stay would be considered for someone that can no longer look after themselves in their own home.

Subacute nursing units – these units provide services that require more intense therapy and/or constant monitoring of the patient. They include intense rehabilitation and a 24-hour licensed registered nurse, (LRN), who is capable of managing the acute and complex problems of the patient. This kind of service is generally considered short-term and, in a rehabilitation center / skilled nursing facility. The patient also has Medicare days, 100 days in fact. How that works is that the first twenty days Medicare will cover the stay at one hundred percent. On day twenty-one that is when the eighty/twenty payment comes into play. Most Skilled Nursing Facilities and Acute Rehabs will work with the Patient to attempt to get them out by day twenty so the patient will not have a payment to the facility.

Nursing home alternatives:

There is also the option of Adult Day Care, which is used for the patients who suffer from dementia, and who need supervision and medical assistance with their day-to-day activities, e.g. their activities of daily living, (ADLs). Such as the need for help with bathing, going to the toilet, and eating, etc. This may be whilst the primary care worker is in the employment of their own. These assisted living facilities are classed as residential care facilities that currently provide individual rooms with three meals a day also on offer to the patient. They provide activities for senior citizens who can no longer care for themselves at home, but they are not considered as needing 24-hour care and constant supervising from a health professional. The care facilities are sometimes referred to as congregate care or congregate living facilities that do also provide the 24-hour care on-site. They provide help and assistance with medication and personal hygiene. However, these kinds of facilities are prohibited from providing skilled nursing services. And they are currently regulated under a different set of state regulations than this that are governed by the nursing home facility. But if skilled nursing care is required for your parent/s, then this can be offered at these institutes via a separate home health agency. There is also no actual doctor involvement in this type of care plan.

There is another option for a plan of care, and that is a board and care home. These facilities are much smaller than the usual care facility and they are more like a home-like residence for patients who can still live independently. They may provide a room with extra assistance in some activities like managing medication and help with the person's health and hygiene. The services and the fees for each service may vary from one residence to another.

Sheltered housing accommodation is also available through the housing and urban development. These kinds of programs may be supplemented by a social worker who is involved in the care of the patient. Workers will help with daily activities if requested, and they have special coordinators and personal care assistants that may help with making meals and taking your parent/s to appointments and personal visits to the family, etc.

There is also the option of continuing care retirement communities, (CCRCs). These facilities may have all levels of living arrangements that are likely to range from independent living to full-time nursing home care.

Another recent initiative is the program of all-inclusive care for the elderly, (PACE). This kind of care is available in some U.S. states. The main aim of PACE is to help the elderly by offering residence to those who meet the requirements for a nursing home placement but are capable of looking after themselves without the constant need for assistance. PACE is a government-run program that basically utilizes a medical and social model of elderly care.

Hospice care is another option if the time is now for your parent/s to get that extra help in their time of need. Hospice care is a special program for patients who are seriously ill or dying. It is a kind of palliative care and it is meant for people who have six months or less to live. The hospice involved in the care of your parent/s will aim to ease the pain of their illness, make the patient/s as comfortable as possible in the last months of their lives. And provide help and support for family members in their time of grief. This kind of care program tries to provide the best possible quality of life for extremely ill and dying patients, and they can do a great job in easing the patient/s suffering. Hospice care is done through a holistic approach, which also offers emotional, mental, physical and spiritual comfort to patients and their close family. The hospice team of carers is a group of people who are well trained and they understand the specific goals of what hospice care is all about, and they really do provide a quality care service for those in need. The hospice team will do their very best to help patient/s live out their final days with dignity, and they will help family members to try to cope with the loss of their loved one. The hospice team of carers can include:

Well-trained and experienced doctors and nurses
Spiritual counselors
Home health aides
Social workers
A mixture of other helpers and volunteers
Bereavement counselors

Hospice care can be provided for your parent/s, and the care can be given wherever your parent/s plan to spend their final days. That may include, in the comfort of their own home, or at a hospital, or in a nursing facility, or in a local hospice facility. Hospice care can truly help the patient/s, and family and friends by providing help and support, education, and counseling. There are numerous services included in hospice care:

Offering spiritual and emotional support for patient/s and their family and friends.
Providing 24-hour care.
Training family members in certain aspects of nursing care to help them to help their parent/s.
Providing speech, physical, and occupational therapies.
Providing help with practical matters including wills, finances, end-of-life directives, and terminal illness awareness / coping strategies.
Managing pain and other symptoms.
Making sure the patient takes their medication.
Coordinating care with the patient/s family doctor and other important health appointments.
Offering bereavement support to family and friends after death.

Whatever your choice of care for yourself or for your parent/s there is always going to be concerned about costs and payments to the nursing home facility that you choose. Payments can quickly increase if the level of care increases. If the person who is entering the nursing facility has come their directly from a hospital and has the Medicare coverage that is needed to cover the costs then it will not be such an issue that creates serious concern. However, Medicare will only pay for a certain amount of time in a care facility. When the financial resources that are available via Medicare are spent, the patient and/or the POA may be liable to cover the rest of the cost of care. This is especially the case if the patient has income and certain assets that will pay for their care facilities.

Will my Medicare pays for hospice care?

An old Hospice Nurse told me "Hospice will allow you to do what you do best and that is to love the Patient."

As we have discovered, hospice care basically refers to a care strategy that is adopted after the patient has been officially certified as terminally ill. And rather than focusing on treating and/or curing the illness, hospice's and the care that they provide is intended to maximize the patient's comfort more than anything else. It is a multi-faceted service which also offers other resources like spiritual and emotional therapies for the patient and their family members. Hospice care is usually administered at the home of the patient, but it can be offered in a hospice unit.

Medicare does provide cover for hospice care to its beneficiaries. And no additional co-payments and/or deductibles are required by the patient for this kind of service. It is covered by the Medicare Part A plan, although the medication side of the service is not covered under Part D. beneficiaries may have to pay a very small fee for their medication to be administered by hospice care staff. However, Medicare coverage does pay for respite care. This care refers to the temporary home or lodging care the patient receives form hospice staff. In some case, the patient may have to pay up to 5% of the respite care charge. When hospice care is accepted, then Medicare will not cover the cost for treatments of a terminal illness, nor will Medicare offer coverage for ambulance transportation and A&E visits, unless each visit is an unrelated illness to the terminal illness. Medicare will pay for numerous health care services, but it may only provide limited payments for nursing facilities. Long-term payments are not considered necessary unless the patient has taken out long-term nursing care insurance with that future concern in mind. Therefore it is wise to read the small print on your Medicare coverage plan/s to be certain if these payments are included. The premiums for this type of long-term cover can also seriously increase your insurance payments to Medicare, so be sure that you have considered all the option available to you when deciding whether or not to purchase long-term health insurance and nursing home coverage. There are many aspects that may need particular attention when considering care home facilities and the other alternative options. But you should definitely consider and/or pay attention to the following:

Research and fully understand all of the different kind of nursing home care and facilities that are available to you, and/or your parent/s

Constantly review your parent/s needs, and also your own ability to provide care for them.

Learn all about your local nursing home facilities, and the services that they provide.

Choose the home that is best for you and your parent/s. Nowhere is absolutely perfect, but with a little effort from yourself, you may just find the ideal facility to provide future care to your parent/s.

Discuss your current situation with medical staff, family and friends, and especially your parent/s to ensure that they are happy with their new set of circumstances.

When visiting nursing homes take in the environment – do they stink of urine? It may be the case that the particular care facility is understaffed, or there is a blatant lack of care at that establishment.

Cheap help does not mean great care – you should shop around and look for the best service that will aid your parent/s in their time of need. Everyone would like to save money but going for the cheapest possible care may result in poor care for your mom or dad.

Try your very best to learn how to deal with your parent/s illness. By being more aware of their symptoms and reactions, etc, you will be able to cope with certain issues regarding their illness, and you will be able to help them when they are suffering. Research your parent/s illness and learn as much as you can about it. By doing so, you will be capable of providing quality care that your parent/s will appreciate.

Providing help and implementing care practices for elderly parents is the role that many people may find quite difficult. And for those that are from older generations, it may mean having to give up a large degree of their personal independence, alongside the issues associated with the feeling like they can no longer play their life-long role of parenthood. It can be extremely difficult for some folk to accept. And for the adult who has to take on the responsibilities of caring for their parents, it can be hard to cope with and hard to even come to terms with too. However, there are many steps that an individual with this added responsibly can take to help minimize the problem and ease their growing concerns.

One of the first steps to implement whilst caring for a parent is to take time out for yourself. Because it is very easy to become totally engrossed in the role of a parental carer. This is understandable as making sure that your loved one is properly cared for, and happy with the care they are receiving is paramount. Keeping your parent in good health is the main role of a carer, but it is also very easy to forget about your own needs whilst trying to ensure your parent/s health and safety in their time of need. Most carers who look after their parents also have to hold down full-time jobs, and they may still have children to care for too. These issues can cause more stress on the process and management of day-to-day life for all concerned. It is okay to put other people's needs before your own occasionally, however, it really should be for a short period, because over time you will quickly find that your own needs are constantly not being met. And it may be time to start thinking about finding extra help with the caring process. Every person needs a break now and then, so before that person becomes completely overwhelmed by their caring responsibilities they should figure out certain ways to take time out and time for themselves. Maybe a short holiday or employing a healthcare nurse would suffice. Maybe searching for a private care company would ease the pressure. These companies can provide live-in care whilst the main carer is on a break if that is what is needed. Private live-in care can provide complete peace of mind for the individual and for those other family members who help to care for your parent/s. it is a care option that can be tailored to meet your loved one's exact requirements, i.e. the person in charge of care can request a nurse who is experienced with Alzheimer or dementia patients, etc.

The next step would be to make a complete lifestyle and care plan. Many carers can fall into the job of being a carer without actually creating a plan of action as soon a sit becomes apparent that one or even both of their parents are in dire need of regular care and lifestyle assistance. The individual carer should assess all options that are available to them and their parent/s, and then discuss all concerns with other family members to find the correct workable care solution for all.

Obviously arranging a power of attorney is a very important step and it should be done immediately. Many elderly parents cannot take care of their finances because of their current condition. Therefore the main carer should be a legally binding financial adviser to deal with all their banking transactions. Not to mention that there are come nasty con men out there who can easily trick your parents into giving away their hard-earned life-savings, so becoming the legal POA will safeguard against any trickster of that kind. Also, people who suffer from dementia may quite easily become slightly confused about their finances and may develop crazy spending habits, so having the legal ability to take control of your parents' financial aspects will put you and your family in a good position to avoid any unwanted and unneeded financial losses.

Another step for a carer to take is to ask family and friends for help in the care process and maybe think about offering them the opportunity to take your parent/s out for the day to ease the strain on your behalf. Your parent/s will also feel the benefit of spending time with others. And it will help keep stress levels to an absolute minimum.

The care of elderly parents can be a massive source of stress due to frustration and other conscious circumstances. And it is absolutely vital that you as the care be completely honest with yourself and others about your feelings. Built up tension will only seriously affect you emotionally. Then it may be you that needs the care from others, because you may suffer some sort of breakdown if you bottle everything up and keep it in without sharing the way you feel. You may even find it very helpful if you discussed your feelings, and about the care process of your parent/s with a doctor or other medical health professional. Especially if you are feeling very low and extremely tired from all the effort that you are making with your parent/s. And if you are suffering from sleeping difficulties, or lack of eating, and /or difficulties in managing your own life, then it is time to speak out about it and to search for extra health care help with caring for your parent/s. you may become increasingly unhappy and stressed out about your current situation, but the best thing to do is not to give yourself such a hard time and to realize the great qualities that you possess because not everyone has the qualities that it takes to be a full-time carer of their parent/s.

The care and the love and support that you give to your parent/s may be easy to offer if you can care for them at home. But you may also feel that putting your mom or dad, or even both of them into a care home is the only alternative that is open to you, because of other concerns and commitments, etc. If that is the case, then you can start by searching for a good care home via your local authority for help.

They will assess your parent/s needs and create a financial plan/options of assistance via Medicare, etc, that is appropriate to your current financial circumstances. You and/or your parent/s may qualify for government assistance but if for some reason you or they do not, then there is no need to worry because you could still ask your local authority in your U.S. state for extra help. They will likely offer as much help as possible to assist you in the care process. You may even want to consider receiving in-home care from a private company that offers a specialized care service for elderly patients. Care at home services will also provide support ranging from a few hours per day up to a 24-hour seven day a week service if that is what is wanted.

Employing a full-time carer will certainly relieve you from a lot of stress and frustration, and it will provide your parent/s with the opportunity to form a relationship with someone outside the close family circle. An extra companion can do your parent/s a world of good. And having a healthcare professional on a daily service may mean that you could continue to enjoy a quality standard of independent living whilst your parent/s are well looked after by someone that is in the know. In-home care can offer shopping services, cooking, social events, and many other services that will help to make yours and your parents live much easier. It is a fact that most elderly people prefer to stay at home whenever possible because they are so used to their own home surroundings, and thanks to this great in-home service that offers quality help and support be experienced and dedicated health caregivers, it is an option for an increasingly higher number of elderly folks choice. It enables them the chance to experience a much better quality of life and within the comfort of their own home instead of a care facility.

There may come a time when you begin to realize that your parent/s are not able to live at home anymore. Old age and related issues or illnesses such as Alzheimer's and dementia can create rising concerns about their health and safety. These types of illnesses can be a constant worry if you are the sole carer of your parent/s. But you still may not want them to reside in a care home or another residential form of care. That is when in-home care will be a great option to assure that your parent/s are still by your side and receiving the best available care that suits their needs. Individual care really can be a quality service that will make yours and your parents that much easier than it would be if it was you alone taking on full care responsibility. We as people work hard throughout our daily lives to try and build a lifestyle that suits us and meets our needs. And we value our independent living, just as our parents have always done. But sometimes it may be best for all concerned if your parent/s were to be put in a residential care unit to help them recover from certain illnesses or just to help them cope with illnesses like dementia which can be very debilitating, and with the extra help always on hand via healthcare professionals in a care home, their everyday lives can be more accommodated in such a place with such well-trained people caring for them.

If you think that your parent/s would be better off in a care facility to help them to cope with their illnesses then that is what you should do. For many people, it simply is not possible for them to have their parent/s at home. Either there is too little space and the home is nowhere near practical enough to care for another person. Or, there are certain work commitments meaning nobody can care for the parent whilst the individual is at work. Then it is time to think and act responsibly and to admit your parent/s into a quality care facility. And once you do that, it is wise to give them some time to settle into their new surroundings, and also give yourself some time to get used to the new circumstances. The worst thing that you could do is to take them home after they have been admitted into a care facility because that can be very dangerous for the patient. For them to be in the care facility it means that health professionals agree with that, and the patient does indeed need extra care and attention. Therefore it would not be safe to take them home just because you are missing your parents, or they are missing you. Standing firm is the best option because in time both you and your parent/s will settle and begin to get used to the new set of circumstances and it could turn into a good situation for everyone concerned. Healthcare professionals understand the many different issues and concerns that families may have over the care of their elders. And they will work with you to make sure that the best possible care package is being delivered to you and your parent/s. All health appointments will be met by using a care facility as they will oversee all doctor's appointments and make sure that the patient is constantly taking their medication.

If a quality care facility is needed to properly care for your parent/s then the first thing to do is make sure that the facility you choose is indeed a QUALITY care facility. There are many signs of a good care facility that provides a quality service. And some important issues and things to be aware of, and to certainly look out for include:

First things first – use your senses.

1. Sight – how do the staff treat their patients? Do they leave the patients in the hallway? How and when do they feed the patients? Is the place clean?

2. Hearing – can you hear patients yelling when you visit the facility? Listen to the care facility nurses, do they speak highly of the place and of their patients?

3. Smell – does the facility smell of urine? Or does it smell unhygienic in some other way?

4. Taste – when you visit the facility try a meal, does it taste nice? Can you bring food into the care facility for your mom and/or dad? Some facilities will allow you to try one.

Another important factor to look out for when you are searching for a quality care facility for your parent/s is to look at the last state inspection that the care facility had. That will tell you most of the important need-to-know stuff about the care home. Every care facility worth its salt will have a current inspection document, and they will be regularly visited by healthcare professionals in different fields who are working to make the facility even better than it already is. The best of the best care facilities will actually allow the patients' families to do what they do best, and that is to take care of their parent/s whilst they are also in receipt of professional help. Before you make any decisions, it is very important to talk to your parents and to be very open with them at all times, as we have already covered in a previous chapter. But you should always plan with them before anything is to happen and yours and your parent/s current situation so you can both be ready for any change of circumstances. Then you can love and support each other throughout the entire care process.

Using Medicare to get a second opinion on your parent/s current health condition:

It is possible to use your Medicare coverage to receive a second opinion from a health professional concerning your parent/s illness and the care that they have been deemed to need. Maybe a physician has recommended a very expensive, or even a very dangerous operation/procedure, you can legally search for the second opinion at a different surgery. Medicare will certainly pay for a second opinion. Because even qualified doctors can make mistakes, and/or make a wrong diagnosis. Medicare Part B coverage will cover the cost for this process, it is even possible to apply for a third opinion from a private firm and Medicare will cover the cost, but a second opinion is usually enough for the patient to accept the diagnosis that has twice been given.

Sadly, nobody lives forever and the time will come when you have to start the process of grieving the sad loss of your parent/s. You must try to grieve and bereave as best you can. This is sure to be one of the saddest moments, but you must begin the grieving process to eventually overcome it. You may grieve forever, however with time the pain of the loss of your parent/s will get easier. Bereavement is the process of grieving and eventually trying to let go of a loved one who is sadly deceased. Family care will go on for some time after the death of a loved one, and the family and friends of the deceased will have to try and cope through what are very difficult times together. But sticking together and helping each other to cope and to grieve is an important part of the bereavement process that must be done for people to move on with their lives. Life does go on after the death of a loved one. So, it is time to grieve and bereave the sad passing of your parent/s and move on to positive thoughts and by thinking positively then you will create positivity in your life. Bereavement is the state of loss that must be overcome after the death of someone close. Many people may be affected by the loss. But you must also concentrate on number one and help yourself to cope with the grief and to finally overcome it and overcome it as quickly as you can before it will seriously affect other important aspects of your life.

The death of someone that is very loved is one of the greatest sorrows that can occur in life. The bereavement process can also accompany other losses, like a decline in your own health and mental well-being. but the grief you are experiencing is very normal because it is actually a healthy response to loss. Everyone, no matter who they are or how tough they think they might be, they will feel helpless in times of grief. That is very normal too, and they must try to cope with the passing of a loved one in their own way. This way may change frequently as there are different stages to the process of the morning. First, the individual must recognize and realize the loss. And the process goes on until the loss of a loved one is eventually accepted.

There is a wide range of emotions that will come across as symptoms after the loss of someone who is close to you, especially the loss of a parent who has looked after you and stood by your side throughout your entire life. Health professional has stated that there are five main reactions to a loss of a parent, and these reactions are in no particular order, and they may even occur at the same time as each other in the person. They include:

Anger and blame

Denial, disbelief, and numbness

The depressed mood with crying and lots of sadness

Feelings of helplessness

Acceptance by coming to terms with the loss

Many people who are grieving will often report a deep sadness with uncontrollable sadness and bouts of depression. Some reports a lack of sleep and that they are unable to be or fell productive any more, be that at home or at work. But eventually these feelings will be overcome and the initial shock from the loss of a parent will ease, and the shock and/or the denial of a loss will be firmly replaced by feelings of anger for some, this anger may be directed at the doctors and nurses or even at family members and/or friends of the deceased. Then the bereavement process may change again, this time with strong feelings of guilt. The person grieving may start to feel as though they could have done more for the parent/s, etc. such feeling and thoughts are very common amongst people, we are all human after all. However, we all should realize that these are simply stages of grief, and everyone deals with grief differently. We must let ourselves and others to grieve and try to complete the bereavement process in their own way. Many may have mood swings and can become quite difficult to deal with, but we must try to bide our time and help those who are struggling to handle and cope well during the grieving process.

Grief may be experienced in lots of different ways including mental, physical, emotional, and social. And the entire bereavement process may depend on the actual relationship with the person who has died.

It may depend on their attachment to each other. The grief of this kind may be described as the presence of a physical or mental illness. Mourning is something that we all must do at some stage of our lives. And it helps us to change and to adapt to a new way of life without the person who has sadly died. If you feel that you are not coping particularly well with your loss and you start to feel seriously stressed out mentally and run down physically, then it is very important that you seek help from your doctor or even a mental health counselor. Albeit, in this time of grief it may seem a lot easier to bury your pain deep inside your mind, but that will only cause more problems both mentally and physically. You must try to face your pain and to talk about it with someone that may be able to help ease your suffering. Be that simply a friendly face with counseling skills or from visiting a doctor who may provide certain medication that will help to calm you down and resolve your emotions. Your reaction to the loss of a loved one will change over time. The death of a parent can be very difficult but you must try your very best to stay strong and eventually to move on. Your parent/s would not want you to remain in a state of grief for the rest of your life. I am sure that they have always wanted the very best for you and grieving for some time is not the best of things to do. It will affect you physically and mentally, it will only keep bringing you down and it may even put a strain on family life as well as your social and working life too.

No matter what age you are currently at in your life, it is sure to be a very sad loss. Losing your parent/s will still deeply affect you as a person and at any age. When your mom or dad dies it could possibly be one of the most emotional times that you have ever experienced. And it is only natural that you may feel consumed by different feelings associated with the pain of a loss of someone that has had such a significant impact/influence in your entire life. When you lose your parent/s it may also feel like you have just lost your lifelong friend as well. It is usual to feel all alone after the passing of your parent/s. however, you must realize as soon as humanly possible, that you are definitely not all alone. There is always someone that can help you, and someone that can show you love and support through these very difficult times. There is also a period of loss that is known as the secondary loss stage. This stage is when you may begin to have many thoughts about all the upcoming experiences that your mom and/or dad can no longer share with you. Things like watching the grandparents growing up, and watching you personally accomplish certain achievements in your future. It is quite possible after the loss of your parent/s that you may start to contemplate your own mortality. This is another normal stage of the grieving and bereavement process. Allowing yourself to grieve and bereave over the loss of your parent/s will help you to say goodbye and say it in your own way. It is all a process, coping with the loss of your mom and/or dad certainly is not an easy task. But with the correct coping strategies in place, you will finally recover from your sad loss.

Anticipatory grief:

Another part of the bereavement process is anticipatory grief. And it is completely normal as it is just a different way to mourn. Anticipatory grief occurs when you are expecting the death of your parent/s or a close loved one. This stage of the bereavement process has many symptoms that are the same as after the death of a parent. Anticipatory grief can include bouts of mild to severe depression that contains extreme concern for and about the person who is likely to die soon. It is a grief that prepares you for death. And it involves the adjustment to change caused by the painful loss of a loved one. This type of grief can give the family of the person who is expected to be soon deceased, it can give them a certain amount of time to come to terms and accept the reality of the impending death of a relative. Anticipatory grief an also give you time to say your goodbyes to your loved one and to tell them how much you love them and how much you have appreciated their help throughout life. People do not feel the same sort of grief before death than they do after death. But also, that experience does not mean that the death will be easier to accept after it happens. However, it may make things a little easier to accept. To accept the death of your parent/s before they have actually died may sound a bit unrealistic, but it does happen to some people who have been caring for their parent/s for some time and have been informed by a health professional that they are terminally ill and to expect the worst. And expecting and accepting the loss of your parent/s can make you come closer together before the sad loss happens. It can make your family and friends attachment stronger too, by helping you and your family and friends to be there for your loved one in their time of need. This may make you all a much stronger unit, and the parent will feel good to see you all together staying strong through what is a very difficult time. Saying goodbye to your parent/s or another close loved one is never easy, but expecting and impending death does provide family and friends with the opportunity to be there for the parent, and it presents them all with the chance to tell them how much they are loved and how much they always will be even after they pass.

Treatments and grief related resources after the death of your parent/s:

Grief as we all know it is a very powerful emotion. It can be very painful and it can be extremely exhausting. And grief can sometimes seem a lot easier to try our best to avoid it instead of confronting grief head-on. But that approach is not really the viable approach if you are searching for a long-term solution. Because burying your grief can only make it manifest in a different area of your life. It can manifest into a physical and/or mental health problem if you do not confront it as soon as possible, and you must try to accept it and come to terms with the loss of your parent/s. It is the only viable route forward. Working and/or even fighting through your sorrow by allowing yourself to accept and express your feelings will be an eventual factor in helping you to heal from the deep wound that is a parental loss. This fighting your grief, or 'grief work' may include a lot of the stages of grief for you the mourner to satisfy your grieving needs, and to help you to complete the bereavement process before you can fully resume your daily life. These stages are all part of the grieving process and it may include trying to separate yourself from the parent who has died. It is a readjustment practice. You have to try to adjust to a world without your mom or dad in it. You must try to form new relationships and build on the ones that you already have. This readjustment stage will only make you stronger. To separate yourself from the parent/s who has recently died you must try to find another viable way to redirect your emotions and other built-up energy that the sad loss has created. It is also very important not to start to neglect yourself whilst you are grieving. Trying to remain focused on yourself in this sad time may be difficult but that is exactly what you should do. Try to eat on a regular basis healthy meals will give you the energy that you need to help you to grieve. The grieving process is extremely tiring, and it can exhaust you both physically and mentally. Experiencing the loss of your mom and/or dad may also remind you of past losses or recent separations. It can have a negative effect on your entire life if you were to let it. You must try to turn that negativity into positivity. Be positive in the thing that you do, think positive as much as you possibly can. You are mourning, so let it be, but be positive.

Mourning may be described as having three different phrases which include:

The constant urge to bring the parent/s who have died back into your life

A deep sadness quickly followed by disorganization of your life

Reorganization of your thoughts and your lifestyle

Mourning can also lead to depression. But much can be done to combat depressive thoughts and we will cover that in the next chapter. However, there are certain treatments that you can personally use such as formal treatments with a health professional and/or support groups, etc. if you feel like you or someone close is experiencing severe difficulties in coping with the sad loss of a parent or other loved one, it is very important that you or they seek professional help. There is always someone to offer their shoulder or ears in your time of need. A family physician can help, or even those health care workers who were looking after you ill parent/s may be a great source of consolation and/or positivity. Even grief therapy or professional counseling may be needed for you to fully recover from the loss. Grief counseling can help you with coming to terms with the reactions of grief, and it will offer you love and support through the grieving process. This form of counseling can be offered via professionally trained personnel or you can visit self-help and support groups in your local area. Bereaved people offer support to each other in such support groups. The services that will offer bereavement support are plenty in each and every state in the U.S. and they may be available in an individual or group setting. The goals of these grief counseling and support services will include the following:

Helping bereaved people to come to terms with their loss by identifying and expressing their feelings related to the loss.

Describing the normal grieving process and all of its stages and encouraging people who are bereaved to accept the loss by talking on an individual or group basis.

Helping the bereaved to fully understand their coping strategies and implementing coping techniques.

Helping the bereaved to separate themselves emotionally from the deceased.

Helping the bereaved to live and to make independent decisions without the deceased.

Describing the differences associated with the grieving processes. i.e. individual grief.

Helping the bereaved to identify coping problems and the certain issues it may cause.

Helping the bereaved overcome their grief by offering continuous support.

Grief therapy can really help those who have lost their parent/s and it is used for those who have more serious reactions to grief. The goals of this particular kind of grief therapy are to help the person identify and to solve the problems/issues that they are currently having due to the separation from their parent/s. When separation issues occur in the person, it may appear as a physical and/or behavioral problem. It could include delayed grief and/ or extreme mourning over the parent/s. It may even include conflicted and extended grief. So the mourners should combat this grief by talking about the deceased and try to recognize the experiences that they are having emotionally because of the loss. The grief therapy may offer the mourner with the opportunity to realize that all their emotions are natural to loss. The guilt, anger, frustration and other negative and uncomfortable emotions can still exist but they mourner should try to think positive about the deceased, grief therapy can help them to do that. Humans, in general, tend to make strong bonds with family and friends. When these bonds are sadly broken due to death, then it is only natural for us to have a strong emotional reaction to that loss. The person must then try to accomplish certain tasks to help them to accept and complete the grief process. This will include acceptance of the broken bond/ loss, and then living with the emotions and adjusting to life without the deceased. We must try to emotionally separate ourselves to finally accept and overcome the grief process.

In this grief therapy service, there are six main tasks that can be used to help the bereaved to work through and fight off their grief. These tasks include:

Finding effective ways to cope with coping techniques and strategies.

Establishing a continuing relationship even though the person is now deceased.

Developing the ability to experience, express and fully adjust to the pain and implement changes to overcome the feelings of grief.

Staying healthy both physically and mentally.

Developing a healthy perception of the new world around you after the loss.

Re-establishing relationships with family and friends by understanding that others may experience difficulties in expressing their emotions and empathizing with the grief that they are experiencing.

Complicated grief:

There may be certain complications in the grief process. This may come about due to certain unresolved issues form the loss. Grief therapy will also involve coping and dealing with certain blockages to the grieving process. A person who is bereaved must identify with any unfinished business related to the loss and accept that the loss is final, then they must begin to see the bigger picture, which is that their own life must still go on without the deceased.

Complicated grief and the reactions involved in it, requires complex therapies. There may be adjustment disorders that are expressed by depression and / or anxiety. This type of complicated grief is identified by the extended time that it takes the individual to overcome their grief. Certain complicated symptoms may also intensify due to this type of grief. It is basically considered unresolved grief, delayed grief, conflicted grief, and / or chronic and acute grief. Grief reactions that may be considered as complicated may also turn into a major depressive disorder that requires urgent treatment. It may also entail post-traumatic stress disorder. Losing a parent is especially hard to cope with, but avoiding the fact that they have died, and avoiding it for some time may result in these types of anxiety disorders.

People have become more aware about mental health and the certain issues it causes for those suffering from mental illness. This is because the stigma associated with mental health is slowly being lifted and we are now prepared to accept the presence of these illnesses in society without discrimination. Providing knowledge about mental health issues and the conditions involved with mental health is extremely important to help fully inform others about it, and with helping those who suffer from mental illness to accept, cope with, and recover from their current issues. Mental health issues like depression can be very difficult to diagnose due to the numerous ways they can manifest. But stress-related illnesses are very common, and many people can suffer in silence without ever seeking help to relieve the symptoms that are causing them so much trouble in their life, both mentally and physically. The stigma behind mental health is making some people afraid to seek help and advice from even their friends and / or family, not to mention seeking help from a professional mental health therapist.

Many people suffer from mental health issues throughout their lifetime due to anything from personal struggles, social isolation, family issues and bereavement. This could be due to the loss of their parent/s, and some people continue their struggle for the rest of their lives while some can quickly recover from the loss and move on quite quickly. They seem to look on the bright side of life no matter what their inner pain may be. And they can simply pick themselves up, dust themselves down, keep calm and carry on. How do some do this and how do others find it more difficult to cope with a sad loss like the loss of a parent? Firstly, it is wise to realize that no matter what their current struggles are, life goes on and it can get better if you try to make it better. Then, it is about acceptance, people can overcome their difficulties and progress to a happier self if they can fully accept their current situation and work on ways to be more productive in their life to improve their current circumstances. Although they might be facing difficulties in their life at the present moment they realize that the difficult times will not last forever and they develop the skills to make the improvements that are needed for a happier self and a happier life. Their thought process is always positive therefore they can quickly overcome the negativity of the struggle that is the loss of their mom and / or dad, and they do this by applying mindful techniques to help them to advance and to recover from their grieving difficulties.

This is because thoughts in general are directly related to a person's positivity and to their current happiness. If you choose to turn a negative thought into a positive thought, it will eventually create a positive result and you will experience a much happier you in the process, even if it is at a time of great loss and inner sadness.

Emotional intelligence is our ability to identify, understand and manage or control our feelings of grief and with emotional intelligence we can additionally perceive, understand and influence our own thoughts. People can improve their emotional intelligence if they practise the techniques that enable them to do so. One way is to observe yourself experiencing an emotion and analyze it in a self-reflection capacity without trying to change the feeling even if it is a negative emotion like guilt, fear or loss. You basically accept the emotion without fighting against it but trying your best to control the pain it causes by making positive counteractive statements in your defense until the guilt, fear or loss subsides and eventually fails to exist in your mindset. This kind of emotional intelligence is directly linked to your thought process and it will certainly help you to come to terms with the loss of your parent/s, and eventually overcome the great grief that you currently feel. Because emotional intelligence is knowing that mastering the self is the first step towards controlling your thoughts, feelings and actions to certain emotions related to death, and this inner intelligence helps with creating effective long-term change that can eventually lead to personal happiness after the loss of a parent. Of course it is not an easy process to recover from such a sad loss, but with emotional intelligence it can become an easier process.

There are always people that can be far too self-critical of themselves and they are constantly scrutinizing by criticizing their every emotion, every thought and every action in a very negative manner. They use their inner-voice to only pinpoint their current weaknesses which only provokes self-doubt, lowers the person's self-esteem and stops them from fulfilling their true potential due to certain self-confidence issues arising from negative thinking. But if they can learn to fully appreciate themselves, they will find the confidence and personal assurance that enables them to beat the blues that being self-over-critical causes internally, it will lead to a happier mindset with a potential for a happier life that they can be proud of. Everybody has weaknesses but if they can find the courage to truly believe in themselves after the loss of their parent/s, then they will open their mind to the opportunity it brings to find their own kind of personal happiness after they have dealt with that loss. It eventually creates the building blocks for inner-strength and self-confidence that will further enable them to concentrate on the awareness of their new-found skills and talents that they hold. Each person in society is capable of great accomplishments if they can strengthen their beliefs and recognize their qualities. Death should not bring the person to feel as though they will never recover from their loss. We should all confront it and accept it as a way of life. We can recover from anything if we are positive. A parental loss is devastating, but we can recover quickly if we change the negativity surrounding the loss into positivity. Positivity about the great life we have shared with our parent/s. etc.

Placing positivity in and throughout your life is liberating. If you can develop a positive mindset you will ensure that the negativity in your life does not corrupt your mind which may lead to certain mental health issues, especially when you are suffering from such a devasting loss. Negative thoughts gradually corrupt the mind in a way that can have an adverse effect on your behavior and attitude towards your own life. A positive thought process will enhance your thinking pattern and help you to become more productive in every aspect of your life. If you can shut out the negativity by counteracting it with a positive mentality you will acquire a freedom that may help to enlighten your entire life and help you to find your happiness after your recovery from grief.

Positivity in life after such a sad loss is your way forward. Negativity is troublesome, and it will only cause you problems in your personal, working and social life. There is no need for you to be stuck in a rut or to be unhappy if you can cancel out the negative by applying positive thinking you will break the vicious cycle and start to aim and look forward to a brighter future after the loss of your parent/s. You can do anything in life if you set your positive mindset towards helping you to recover from the bereavement and then go on to achieve your life goals. Positive thinking makes you stronger after parental loss and it will create opportunities that you may not have realized were possible due to the negativity taking over certain aspects of your life. Attack the negativity that is restricting you form your recovery from grief with a newfound positivity and you will succeed in breaking free and committing to change. Furthermore, if you can build strong, positive and healthy relationships with the rest of your family and friends after such a loss it can then supply you with the foundation to break free from your current mindset and work towards initiating optimism for the future instead of a long drawn out grieving process, and it can fill you with a sense of well-being that will lead to change and provide you with the potential for future happiness.

If you struggle too, or you feel that you cannot possible overcome the grief that is associated with the loss of your parent/s, then you will eventually succumb to certain mental health issues that you will need to address. These illnesses can include both depression and anxiety disorders as well as many other grief related illnesses.

Depression - (major depressive disorder) is a common and serious medical illness that negatively effects how people feel and affects the way they think and how they may act. Fortunately, depression is also a very treatable disorder with certain medication and practises to help reduce the depressive thoughts and the actions that are associated with it. Depression can cause feelings of sadness and / or a severe loss of personal interest in certain activities that the person may have once enjoyed. It can lead to a variety of emotional and physical problems that can seriously decrease a person's ability to function, be it, at work or at home. Symptoms of depression can include:

Feeling sad and/or having a depressed mood

Loss of interest or pleasure in activities once enjoyed

Changes in appetite – weight loss or gain unrelated to diet

Trouble sleeping or sleeping too much

Loss of energy or increased fatigue

Increase in purposeless physical activity (e.g. hand-wringing, pacing or slowed movements and speech (actions which are observed by others)

Feeling worthless and/or guilty

Difficulty thinking, concentrating or making decisions

Thoughts of self-harm and/or contemplation of suicide

Most people have minor ups and downs in mood (mood swings) when they feel good one day but then they feel very low the next. These changes in mood often have an identifiable cause such as the sad loss of a parent, or close family member, etc, and they can last for quite some time or even pass very quickly. Depression is associated with physical symptoms that include the above. In some cases, a depressive illness follows a traumatic event in a person's life, such as divorce, bereavement, or the loss of a job. In other cases, it follows a time of major life change, such as retirement or death of a close loved one. It may also be precipitated by hormonal changes at the menopause stage or even after childbirth. However, in many cases, depression has no apparent cause, and some people suffer repeated episodes throughout their lifetime.

There are other forms of depression which include anxiety disorder:

Anxiety – Experiencing occasional anxiety is a normal part of life. However, people with serious anxiety disorders frequently have intense, excessive and persistent worry and fear about everyday situations. These feelings of anxiety and panic interfere with daily activities and they can be difficult to control, most times they are out of proportion to the actual danger they hold and they can last a long time if the person who is suffering is also grieving over the loss of a parent. People suffering from anxiety may avoid places or situations to help prevent these reoccurring feelings of self-doubt. Symptoms may start during childhood or the teenage years and continue into adulthood, and / or after a parent passes. Examples of anxiety disorders include generalized anxiety disorder, social anxiety disorder (social phobia), specific phobias, e.g. crowded places, etc, and separation anxiety disorder. People can have more than one anxiety disorder at the same time. Sometimes anxiety results from a medical condition that needs treatment and it can cause other mental and physical problems linked to stress.

Common anxiety signs and symptoms can include:

Feeling nervous, restless and/or tense

Having a sense of impending danger, panic/doom/paranoia

Increased heart rate

Rapid breathing (hyperventilation)

Sweating profusely

Trembling

Feeling weak or tired

Trouble concentrating or thinking about anything other than the present worry

Sleeping difficulties

Experiencing gastrointestinal (GI) problems

Feelings of guilt

Difficulty controlling worry

Having the urge to constantly avoid things/situations that trigger the anxiety

If you are suffering from anxiety from the loss of your parent/s, you will feel apprehensive, tense and unable to concentrate, and unable to think clearly or to even sleep well at night. It may emulate a sense of foreboding for no obvious reason or you may suffer from repetitive worrying thoughts. People also have symptoms such as headaches, sweating profusely, chest pains, palpitations, abdominal cramps and general feelings of tiredness. Anxiety is a natural reaction to daily stress and it is normal to feel anxious if, for example, you are worried about things concerning finance issues or family matters. Such anxiety may help you to deal with stressful events and can help to improve your performance in certain situations, hence, the fight or flight concept in life. However, anxiety is not normal if it is without apparent cause or if it is so severe that you feel as though you cannot cope with everyday life. That is when you must seek professional help to combat anxiety. The loss of your parent/s can manifest into many anxiety and depressive disorders, so help must be found to enable you to cope with the grief.

If you experience any of the above symptoms, then sadly, you are clinically depressed. Being depressed can seriously affect your entire life if you do not find ways to combat your depression. Suffering from depression can be debilitating if not addressed by asking for help and / or by using coping techniques and strategies to reduce the risk of the condition deteriorating, which sometimes can be at a rapid rate. Psychological therapies will help with a person's depression. There are a variety of therapies available, some explore the person's past, while others focus on current behaviour and / or their thought processes due to parental loss. All will involve a therapist who usually encourages the person to talk about their feelings and the fears they have in the lives, and about their deceased parent/s while providing help and advice at the same time. It can include one to one, or group sessions depending on the individual taking therapy. There are many actions that you can take to try to control depression and other associated illnesses, which will be discussed in more detail, but first you must accept that right now, you are not feeling your usual self and that you may indeed be depressed. Realizing this and accepting it will start the process of recovery from your recent bereavement. You are only human therefore you can only do the best you can to understand that you cannot control everything in life, and you certainly cannot control the passing of your parent/s. However, you can control your thoughts about your parent/s and about the bereavement. By giving yourself a break and treating yourself with kindness and understanding, you will move forward and break the heavy chains of depression and become your own best friend in the process of your recovery. Being in a dark place after losing a parent is not a nice place for anyone, but if you slow down and try to take a moment to reflect on your current situation you will finally start to see the light at the end of the grieving tunnel. When you feel stressed remind yourself of how far you have come in life and think of all the good times that life itself has provided you and your parents. If depression continues to show its ugly face, try to confront it with a clear mind. Confronting problems head on is the best way to deal with them, but do not be afraid to tell others and ask for help if you feel that you need it. There are many people who would love to help you in your time of grief, including family and friends or a friendly counselor who will explore options and provide opportunities for recovery by being a shoulder to cry on, and / or by simply being someone to talk too and to express your feelings to without any judgement being passed.

If you are depressed, you should try to avoid stagnation. Remaining stagnant will only cause future problems. When people are depressed they tend to sit around on daily basis doing nothing. This causes added tension both mentally and physically, it also inhibits the flow of energy which has an adverse effect on motivation. Moving around throughout the day allows energy to flow naturally and this extra energy can help to fight against depression. Simple movements will provide beneficial factors that continue to increase with time including the reduction of stress and anxiety caused by muscular tension. It is important that you also use the body to help heal the mind. Albeit, that is not to say that you cannot take time out and relax, but when you do, you should try to activate your mind as well. Keeping your mind active when your body is not will help you to stay motivated towards the end goal of overcoming depression and recovering from the loss of your parent/s. One of the greatest things people have is their imagination. If it is used to their advantage, people are capable of great accomplishments. You can use your imagination as a tool for recovery if you create thoughts of positivity that increase your inner well-being. By simply creating thoughts of prosperity and even grandeur about your future it will focus your mind on possible productivity that may improve your current lifestyle as well as your future. Your imagination is such an effective tool that can create absolute change in your life. You can methodically plan for the future in your imagination and that plan can be full of happiness even after a loss. It is basically called visualization when you enter your mind and start to imagine a new you without your parent/s, a new way of life, a place where you have fully recovered and you no longer feel lonely and isolated. A place where your world is no longer filled with worry off grief.

The most important difference between a person that is depressed and a person who is happy is in their thoughts. A depressed person can look at the same circumstance as a happy person can, or they can even be in the same predicament concerning an issue in their life. However, the depressed person will only look at the circumstance from a negative view while the happy person will see the negative but apply positive thinking to find an opportunity for some sort of personal growth by learning from the issue and implementing practises to ensure a positive situation arises from the negative circumstance.

Despite the difficulties depressive mental illnesses pose, sufferers should never give up hope as depression can be beaten. Many people experiencing a journey of darkness like that associated with parental loss can and do make a full recovery and live happy fulfilling lives. It may take time and different paths may be needed to be taken before the road to recovery from grief can eventually suffice. With the right treatment, counseling, coping strategies and a solid support network in place, everyone suffering with mental health issues after bereavement can eventually move on and they can then transform depression into an experience that makes that individual much stronger and capable of facing, exploring and conquering future life challenges with confidence.

With a positive mindset you can embrace life after loss with fresh creative thoughts and new opportunities by being productive in pursuing your personal happiness. Always reward yourself for your achievements no matter how big or small some may be, they are all accomplishments that are positive, and they may provide you with the extra confidence that is needed to achieve more objectives and personal goals you hold for your own life. Self-appreciation will help to combat and eradicate negativity. It may help you to seek and find the positive even from a negative thought or set of circumstances. Positivity will help you to encounter success if you apply it in your life and maintain a motivation to transform your mind from a negative and depressive thought process. Positivity will inspire you to be in control and contemplate what life can be like for a new happier you.

Overcoming depression after parental loss requires self-analysis and a little help from your family and friends. Making lifestyle changes if your life is stressful and by trying to minimize the harmful effects that stress may cause will help with happiness. Finding time to keep up with your friends and family, taking up leisure activities, exercising regularly, changing habits and finding new hobbies will lead to you being healthier in both body and mind. If you break stressful tasks down into smaller, easier parts it will ease the pressure that you might feel building up in your life because of the loss that you have recently experienced.

If people start to make heavy demands on you, try to set limits to their demands and create the life you want to live on your terms. If you hit another low, accept it and learn from it. You can overcome anything in life when you realize that some things are beyond your control and influence, but you can control your thoughts towards them. Think positive. Treat yourself and your life as a work in progress after the loss and you will develop confidence that will help you to change after acceptance and to finally go out there and reach your life goals. People from all walks of life can find personal happiness if they start with self-recognition. If you recognize your faults, you can learn from them, but better still, if you start to recognize your unique qualities and the opportunities / possibilities that life brings, you will start to grow in self-confidence and with that new self-confidence it will bring a happier, more opportunistic and optimistic you. Start to look on the bright side of life and you will experience personal growth related to personal happiness. Be comfortable as you and continue to appreciate and love yourself because underneath the negative thoughts that you may have is a beautiful person waiting to break free from bereavement with unlimited potential. Be your own cheerleader because you have undoubtedly accomplished some amazing things in life and you will continue to do so if you hold a positive and optimistic mental attitude. But be patient and give yourself the time that is needed to change and to accept the death of your parent/s. Be brave, be proud, be strong, be you and never give up.

Happiness is a perception and it is all about learning to be happy. Understanding how your body / mind works after grieving, and how to look after yourself by combatting and controlling stress-related illnesses due to it is essential if you aspire to stay healthy. Because if you decide to add positivity in your life instead of always focusing on the negativity after bereavement, I am confident that by doing this, everyone can be happier in life and obviously that includes you. If you change your mindset you can change your life. You are the master in command of your own recovery. In psychology, happiness is a mental or emotional state of well-being with positive, pleasant emotions ranging from contentment, amusement, satisfaction, gratification and personal triumph to extreme joy or euphoria, referring to the 'good life'. Fulfilling one's ambitions, reaching one's full potential can make a person happy. Therefore finding happiness after a personal tragedy such as the loss of a parent can be considered as a kind of conditioning. If you train your mind to be positive and you can keep that state of mind throughout life then surely you will be capable of overcoming the grieving process related to personal loss. This does not mean that a positive and a happy mind is immune to other emotions, because other emotions are critical to help a positive mind to cope and to deal with the difficult times. It simply means that a happy / positive mind is much more better equipped to deal with those negative emotions and to learn from them and to combat and overcome their grief.

So how do you train your mind for positivity?

It is about learning from your other emotions that bring unhappiness and negativity and having the capacity and strength of mind to snap back into a happier / positive state of mind after you have dealt with the negative emotions. Most people might say that they know happiness when they experience it. Great thinkers for centuries have deemed that the most fundamental human goal is to be happy.

Your parent/s would certainly want you to be happy and to think positive, and they would certainly want you to recover from your grief and to accept that they have gone. But they would also want you to move on with your own life and to find a way to be happy until one day you may all meet again. Try to be optimistic about your future without your parent/s. It will certainly help you to recover from the grieving process and it will eventually turn the negative into positive.

Optimism is a virtue that can make you recover from the sadness of parental loss, and it can eventually lead to personal happiness. It fills you with an energy that helps you continue to keep moving forward in life after a loss in the family. Even in the face of diversity, obstacles or failures, optimism gives you the momentum to keep pushing forward and to achieve your own goals. Optimism is a form of hope. An optimistic approach to life after a bereavement in the family is what will find you your happiness after the grieving process. This is because it is a mindset that allows us to approach life's challenges without dread. Optimism shows possibility and great potential. It is the key to opening opportunities and to utilizing different options and solutions to certain challenges. Optimism can give you the determination to overcome obstacles and realize your dreams. It allows you to see possible avenues to personal achievement. With optimism you can envision creativity that will help you to get to where you want to be after a long bout of sadness. Happy people in general seem to look at the world optimistically and you can too. It provides you with a better sense of well-being and helps to reduce stress and fear of the unknown related to grief. The benefits of thinking and feeling optimistic are plenty which explains how people consistently strive for success and manage to achieve their set goals. This eventually leads to happiness. Psychological research indicates that optimism allows people to see life's setbacks as learning processes that are useful and worthwhile because it helps them to reach all the targets they set if they have an optimistic attitude towards them. Some successful people even seek out opportunities that they expect to fail in order to get the feedback and information they need as a learning tactic. Optimism is thought to have both psychological and physical health benefits that make those who are optimistic healthier than those who constantly think of life in a pessimistic manner after they have suffered a loss. Therefore, if you are a negative thinker but you want to change your mind set and indeed your life after bereavement, then you should start to think and feel optimistic and it will result in you finding your personal happiness. If you can find a way to cut out the negativity that bereavement has caused and that is wearing you down day by day and eating away at your confidence and happiness, and if you can then replace it with optimistic positivity you can create an improved environment with possibilities that may lead you being happier once you have finally came to terms with your loss of a loved one. Positive thinking with positive and optimistic self-talk and affirmations about how good you feel and how constructive your life is going to be from now and in the future is a great tactic to find happiness after bereavement. If you can transform a negative thought into a positive thought you will improve your perception of yourself and your life in general. Keep feeding the mind with optimism and positivity and it will eventually accept all the suggestions that you decide to offer about yourself. It will become easier to defeat and dismiss thoughts of negativity that are holding you back from moving on with your life. Your parents would have been optimistic about your future throughout theirs and your entire life. So try to make them proud even after they are deceased and you will feel the benefit from the optimism and positive thinking that this creates. Replace negativity with positivity.

To fully recover from the bereavement of your loved one, or to even cope with all of the complications that the caring process brings, especially whilst caring for an elderly parent that is in need of your constant care, you must try to fulfil your own needs to ensure that you can recover completely after the death of a loved one, or to ensure that you are capable of continuing caring for your parent/s. All of your personal needs should be fulfilled to maintain the motivation that is needed to either recover and move on, or to provide you with the strength to carry on caring for your parent/s. Maslow's hierarchy of needs is relevant in finding ways to fulfil your own needs whilst coming to terms with a loss, or whilst caring for elderly parents:

Physiological – Satisfying the person's secondary needs; ensuring health materials and benefits are in place to start recovery. Providing water, breaks, comfortable area to talk, etc.

Safety – Environment clear from hazards and potential danger. All tasks and talks are completed in the correct manner with the person's safety and health in mind always.

Love/belonging – Affiliation; Motivating the person suffering from depression into realising that they are important, and their input is needed to assure steps to change success. Providing a friendly environment that helps the person to feel at ease.

Esteem – Motivational techniques to provide the person with motivation and the want to make changes in their life; Acknowledging their achievements. Reaching targets, objectives and goals. Giving the person suffering the recognition for attaining certain milestones.

Self-actualisation – Cognitive; realisation of the person's potential. Congratulating them on good performance and changes. Satisfying the person's primary needs and providing opportunities for them to realize their accomplishments.

You can see how Maslow's hierarchy of needs is relevant in helping a person to fulfil their personal needs if it is used in the correct way it will change a person's perception of their own life if all the needs in Maslow's theory are met. If your current caring lifestyle is stressful, try to fulfil your needs and you will be on your way to a happier lifestyle and a happier you which is brought on by change. You must continue to fulfil your own needs to enable you to grieve and accept your loss, or to continue caring for your parent/s in a manner that they will appreciate.

Not wanting to end this book talking about loss and needs, we will cover the expected changes to Medicare in 2019. There are to be some important changes that you must be aware of, so we will discover and discuss them in this final chapter.

If you the patient, or your mom or dad is contemplating a change in the Medicare coverage. Then there are some important factors that you need to be aware of. Most importantly, is the fact that changes can only be made at the Open Enrollment Period, (OEP). At this enrollment stage, which is usually occurs each year from October 15th through to December 7th, you can change the following:

You the patient, or your parent/s can join a new Medicare Advantage Plan. Or a stand-alone prescription drug plan, which is Medicare Part D.

You are able to switch between the Original Medicare with or without a Part D plan and Medicare Advantage.

The things that you, or your parent/s should keep in mind whilst you are choosing to change Medicare coverage are:

All changes that are made during the OEP will not take effect until January 1st.

If you or your parents currently have Medicare Advantage, then it is possible for you to also switch to the Original Medicare plan, enabling you to join and receive Part D coverage if you wish to do so.

The OEP is the only occasion that you can are able to choose a new Medicare Advantage or a Part D plan.

Depending on where you live, it may also be possible for you the patient, or your parents to purchase a Medigap policy. This is a policy that helps you to pay the costs for Medicare coverage. Although limitation may apply as to who can actually purchase a Medigap policy.

If, for some reason you, and / or your mom or dad are dissatisfied with the current health coverage that you / they receive. Then you must make the all-important changes at the OEP date. You may be unhappy about your Original Medicare plan, if so, you should regularly check for lower costs and certain beneficial features that might change each year. If you have purchased the Medicare Advantage plan or the basic Part D prescription drug plan, you should receive an Annual Notice of Change (ANOC) and / or you should be provided with Evidence of Coverage (EOC) from the date of any changes made to your Medicare coverage. It is wise to review all of your, or your parents notices from Medicare for any important changes that occur on a yearly basis. Some changes could include many benefits. Cost of coverage may be much lower for next year, and certain rules about each plan may be changed or upgraded for the upcoming year of your Medicare coverage. Even if you are satisfied with your Medicare coverage, it can still be very beneficial to search for more Medicare options in the U.S. state that you or your parents currently reside in. Research has shown that people with Part D Medicare coverage can substantially lower the cost of the plan if they shop around, online and offline for the best possible deal each year.

The best way to enroll in any Medicare plan is to call 1-800-MEDICARE.

Enrolling in a new plan directly via Medicare is certainly the best option to take to fully protect yourself or your parents, if for some reason there is an issue with the enrollment process. By enrolling through Medicare it will ensure that all details are safe, including the date of enrollment, the representative's details who handle the enrollment process for you will be logged, and any backdated coverage that may need to be issued will be received without delay. Remember that when you do enroll in a new plan at the OEP date you must confirm all the Medicare coverage details with plan itself. As of 2019, there are to be some important changes to Medicare coverage. These changes will affect the enrollment process. Medicare Advantage and the Part D prescription drug plan will forego some changes as will Medicare premiums, co-payments, deductibles, and costs. Medicare will announce those changes to their coverage beneficiaries, but this is the expected coverage changes for the year 2019, in which Part A - B – D are forecasted to experience change:

Part A costs in 2019:

Premium – if you or your parents have between 30 and 39 working quarters – total cost - $240 per month

Premium – if you have fewer than 30 working quarters – total cost - $437 per month

Deductible – total - $1364 per benefit period

Inpatient – hospital daily coinsurance for days 61 to 90 – total - $341 per day

Inpatient – hospital daily coinsurance for 60 lifetime reserve days – total - $682 per day

Skilled nursing facility – daily coinsurance for 21 to 100 – total - $170.50 per day

Part B costs in 2019:

Premium – total cost - $135.50

Annual deductible – total - $185

Part B income-related monthly adjustment amount (IRMAA) in 2019:

Individuals earning below or equal to $85.000 annually – total - $135.50

£85.000 - $107.000 – total - $189.60

$107.001 - $133.500 – total - $270.90

$133.501 - $160.000 – total - $352.20

$160.001 - $499.999 – total - $433.40

$500.000 and above this amount – total - $460.50

Part D costs in 2019:

National average premium – total cost - $33.19

Annual deductible – total - $415

Coverage will begin – total - $3.820

Catastrophic coverage will begin – total - $5.100

Part D (IRMMA) costs in 2019:

Individuals earning an annual income below or equal to $85.000 – additional payment to regular Part D – total - $0

$85.000 - $107.000 – total - $12.40

$107.001 - $133.500 – total - $31.90

$133.5001 - $160.000 – total - $51.40

$160.001 - $499.999 – total - $70.90

$500.000 and above annually – total - $77.40

Exclusions form Medicare coverage in 2019:

Medicare will not cover all items and services related to your health care in the year 2019. The items and services excluded from Medicare coverage will be as followed:

Alternative medicines; this includes acupuncture, experimental procedures and certain treatments, and also chiropractic services, except the manipulation of the spine procedures.

Most dental care; dental care will not be covered in Medicare coverage 2019.

Care received outside the United States; most health care received outside the U.S. may not be a part of your Medicare coverage in 2019, however they may be certain exceptions for some.

Hearing aids; this also includes examinations related to prescribing and / or fitting the hearing aid. Albeit, in some cases the implants to treat severe hearing deficiency or loss may be covered in 2019.

Personal care; this also includes help with bathing, eating and dressing the patient in a health care situation.

Non-medical services; including a private hospital room. Hospital television is not included and telephone shave also been taken out of the Medicare coverage for 2019, including copies of x-rays, and health appointment of non-medical emergencies, etc.

Nursing home care; this only applies to long-term nursing home care. The short-term will still be covered by certain Medicare coverage plans in 2019.

Non-emergency transportation; including taxi costs and ambulette services.

Most vision care; this also includes coverage for eye glasses and examinations for prescribing eye glasses, except in the cases of cataract surgery.

You may also be eligible for what is known as DME coverage. This is Durable Medical Equipment. Whether you are currently in receipt of Original Medicare or Medicare Advantage plan. Those Medicare plans will cover your DME needs if you can sufficiently meet the following two conditions:

Your primary health care provider, or (PCP) has signed an order, certificate or prescription after they have had a face-to-face visit with you. In this particular document, your PCP should state that the required office visit between you both actually occurred, and you officially need the DME to help you with your current medical condition, and / or an injury that you have recently received, and that the equipment is needed at your home for your personal use. And that your face-to-face office visit / meeting has taken place no more than six months before the prescription for DME is written.

Once you have received your PCP's order / prescription for your DME, you must then take it to the correct supplier to receive the full coverage. You must be aware and be sure that you only use an equipment supplier who has official approval from your current

Original Medicare or Medicare Advantage plan. However there is a completely different process if the DME is for coverage of a manual or electric powered wheelchair or a scooter.

For vaccines and immunizations / preventative services. Medicare Part D will cover most of the vaccines and / or immunizations that you may need throughout the year. However, there are certain ones that are actually covered by the Medicare Part B plan. These include: Influenza / flu shots – including both the seasonal flu vaccine and the swine flu vaccine.

Pneumonia vaccines – all Pneumococcal shot are covered under Part B.

Hepatitis B shots are also covered under the Medicare Part B plan. The Medicare Part B plan also covers vaccines after you have been exposed to any dangerous viruses and / or diseases. An example of these viruses or diseases are Tetanus shots if you have had an injury from a nail or a rabies shot may be needed if you have been bitten by a stray dog.

You as the Medicare beneficiary are fully responsible for the full costs of care if you currently receive a service that Medicare does not cover. But if you are on the Medicare Advantage Plan, your plan may cover some of the services above, it is always wise to contact your plan provider and ask if your coverage applies to the above and / or any additional items and services.

If your health care provider refuses to file a claim because in certain situations your current health care provider may be unwilling to file your claim or submit a bill for Medicare to cover it concerning your recent health care. You should be aware of the following:

HIV screenings are also provided under Preventative services. HIV attacks the body's immune system and it can quite easily lead to other diseases like AIDS. The screening process can help to determine if you need any treatment for HIV. Eligibility is covered under the Medicare Part B plan and it is an annual coverage.

Your provider may believe that your Medicare will deny coverage of costs. Therefore your provider must ask you to sign what is called an Advance Beneficiary Notice, (ABN). Before you decide to sign this notice, it is wise to ask certain questions to find out whether your current provider considers the service to be officially medically necessary, and to ask them if they will actually help you to appeal if coverage is denied.

You must then still ask your provider to file the claim to Medicare, even if they think that the claim will be denied. Do this because you may still appeal against any decision that is made by your current Medicare coverage plan.

Your provider may even ask you to pay the full bill of your health care services if you are seeing a participating provider, therefore you must ask your current provider to submit the claim to Medicare and they should let you know exactly what you owe in terms of payment after the services have been processed for the claim. It may also help to make direct contact with your medical licensing board to report the issue of concern.

Non-participating providers are also allowed to submit a request for full payment and the payment to be paid upfront at the time of the health care service. It is then wise to ask your current provider to file a claim with Medicare coverage on your behalf. That way you may quickly receive Medicare reimbursements and they could be up to a total of 80% of the Medicare approved amount.

If your current provider has opted out of Medicare, then those opt-out providers have to have signed an agreement to be excluded from the Medicare program and they will have to provide you with proof of that agreement. But it is highly likely that they will not bill Medicare for the care services that you receive whilst in their care, therefore you will be expected to pay the full bill.

You should still submit a reimbursement request form to your current Medicare coverage plan to help you to pay the costs of the care service. Because Medicare may still cover certain costs related to the service from the opt-out provider.

If your current care provider refuses to bill Medicare without informing you why they will not send them the bill. This act is considered a Medicare fraud, and you should report it immediately.

If the current provider still refuses to bill Medicare, then you may want to file a claim against that provider, and to also submit a claim for cover of care costs for yourself. You can do that by submitting a Patient's Request for Medicare Payment form.

Receiving an Advance Beneficiary Notice, (ABN) from your current health provider is quite easy to attain. If you are currently in receipt of the Original Medicare coverage, and your provider has a reason to think that the Medicare plan you are on will refuse / deny coverage for the service they provide because of the Medicare medical necessity requirement/s. They should then give you and ABN to read and to sign if you are happy with it, and for you to receive the care from that particular health care provider. But you must note that you will definitely not receive an ABN if you are currently on the Medicare Advantage plan, so do be aware of that fact. If you were to receive an ABN form your current health provider, then there are also several other things that you should ask them before you decide to choose their service. You should ask them if they think the service they are about to provide is medically necessary. Then you should also ask them if they are willing to help you to appeal by helping you to write a letter describing and justifying your current medical need for the service that they are offering you.

Have you received your new Medicare card for 2019?

Your new Medicare coverage card has a Medicare number that is now unique to you. It is being replaced for Medicare coverage instead of your Social Security number. This has been done to protect your confidential information and it will certainly help to combat against any Medicare fraud. When you receive your Medicare coverage card you should do the following:

Destroy your old Medicare coverage card as soon as your 2019 card has arrived.

Start using your new Medicare coverage card straight away. Take it with you to your doctors and other healthcare institutes as they may ask for your new Medicare number.

Protect your Medicare number like you do with your Social Security number. Only give this number to your current doctor and any health practises / hospitals that you may visit for health care.

Keep all your other plan cards, and always keep in a safe place at all times. You may need to show all of your plan cards when you visit a practise / hospital in the year 2019.

Are you still waiting to receive your Medicare coverage card for 2019?

If you are still waiting to receive your Medicare card, then it really should have arrived in the mail by now as Medicare have been sending the card since April 2018. If for some reason you have not received the card or you have misplaced it, then you should do the following:

Check your mail. You may have simply not realized that the Medicare card has changed and they have issued you with a new Medicare number. The Medicare coverage card will arrive in a white envelope and it will be addressed from the Department of Health and Human Services.

If you cannot find your new Medicare coverage card, then you are welcome to call 1-800-MEDICARE, and they will issue you with a new coverage card as soon as possible.

Until that new card arrives you may still use your old card in case of any emergency health care issues.

How to get the best out of your Medicare coverage:

You can receive help to choose the coverage that best suits your current needs. You can receive free personalized counseling. You can receive this help from the State Health Insurance Assistance program or call 1-800-MEDICARE.

You can receive more free help with any Medicare question that you may have by visiting Medicare.gov, or by again calling 1-800-MEDICARE.

You can also receive preventative services by asking your current doctor or by contacting another health care provider who offers preventative services like screenings and tests. Medicare coverage currently offers many preventative services at no extra cost to the patient.

You can receive more help with paying for your health care by finding out if you are eligible to get help with paying your health and prescription drug costs. You should check your current Medicare plan to see if you qualify for this extra service.

You can now go paperless with your Medicare coverage and with all of the other health plans that you are currently on. You can also help save tax dollars by going paperless and choosing to access future Medicare and You handbooks electronically. It is very easy to access your Medicare coverage plans online.

Are there any other types of Medicare health plans and projects available to you?

There are some types of Medicare health plans that currently provide health coverage that is not part of the Medicare Advantage plans. But they are officially still classed as part of the Medicare coverage system. Some of these plans currently provide Medicare Part A (hospital insurance), and Medicare Part B (medical insurance) coverage. Whilst some may only provide Part B coverage. These different plan coverages have some of the same rules and restrictions related to Medicare Advantage plans. However each type of plan has special rules and exceptions, so you should always make contact with your current plan provider to receive more information and / or to express your interest in any plan that you do not currently receive as part of your Medicare coverage.

There is now Medicare Cost Plans available, and also programs of All-inclusive for the Elderly plans, and many different Medicare Innovation Projects are currently available for you to purchase.

Do you know your rights and how to fully protect yourself from Medicare fraud?

Your Medicare rights are as followed:

You have the right to be treated fairly and with dignity. You should be treated with respect at all times during your Medicare coverage.

You have the right to receive information in a way that is clear for you to understand from Medicare and other health care providers. If you do not understand any information then inform them about it.

You have the right to be protected from any discrimination.

All of your personal and health records should always remain private and confidential.

You have the right to have all of your concerns and questions answered by Medicare and other health providers and / or professionals.

You have the right to participate in any treatment decisions.

You have the right to have access to a doctor and other health care providers, specialists and facilities in your time of need.

You can receive Medicare-covered services in any medical emergency.

You have the right to receive a prescription and to review and / or appeal against any medication that you do not agree with.

You can file a complaint or grievance at any time you wish against Medicare or any other health care organization.

You have the right to receive quality health care.

You have the right to access all of your personal health information at any time.

Your right to access your personal health information at any time is granted by law. Either you or your legal representative on your behalf has the right to view and to receive copies of all of your personal health information and all of the records detailing your health care form your current and / or past health providers. You can access any and all of your health plan records via Medicare at any time you wish. You also have the legal right to have a provider or Medicare health plan to send you copies of all the information that they currently hold about you. And / or any information that they have shared with a third party, which may include other providers who have treat you in the past or recently. Any information that you wish to receive on request should be sent to you as soon as possible after the request.

This information may include:

Information about your Medicare enrollment process and the plans that you are currently enrolled on.

Any claims and / or billing records that you wish to access.

Your medical records from childhood and adulthood concerning you health providers, doctors, hospital visits, etc.

Your medical and your case management records are always available for you to request access to. Apart from your psychotherapy records.

Any other information that you suspect doctors and health professionals hold about you and your health plans.

You may have to fill out a health information request form and to pay a small cost-based fee for Medicare and other health care providers to send you copies of the information they hold about you. But your providers and health plans will inform you about the fees that are involved in sending you copies of the information. Although, in most cases you may not actually have to pay a small fee if you store the information electronically and view it via the process of downloading it or looking at your records online through their own health care portal.

And you have the right to receive all the information that health care providers hold about you in a timely manner. However, your records may take up to 30 days before you do receive them, especially if you have asked for them to be delivered to you by post.

Medicare in particular, will certainly protect all the records and information that they hold about you. It will do its utmost to protect your privacy and your health information.

The Author, Robert Gatewood, is a fourteen-year veteran of the Missouri Army National and the U.S. Navy. When discharged from the military, I started to go to school EMT, Phlebotomy, Certified Nursing Assistant, LPN, and RN. I was inspired to be a nurse by my grandmother Louise Brewer. She went to school with my Aunt Mary Lemay and received their PN at the Decanis School of Nursing in St. Louis, MO. I would spend my summers with my grandmother. She taught me to do a nursing assignment and how to take a blood pressures. When her friends would come over and say they don't feel well. She would have me to do assessments and vital signs. That showed me how to be a nurse.

Per the family history my mother was also a graduate of Decanis School in the X-Ray Program, she had passed away from a car accident in Salt Lake City, UT.

When I was discharged from the military I also wanted to go to Decanis School of Nursing, but to my dismay, it was closed one year before I was discharged from the service. I attended another school in the St. Louis Area. I received a Certificate of Nursing and then Associated Degree in Nursing.

Working in the St. Louis Area in Hospitals and Home Health to pay for school. After being an RN for 2-3 years I was told that I was losing my hearing and was fired from my job at a local hospital. As soon as the door shut behind me my phone rang and it was a recruiter asking if I had ever been a case manager. I said no but, I am now. That is when I started on my path as an RN Case Manager. Working for some talented Directors of CM and Nurses received my ACM Certification in the Summer of 2018.

I currently have been working as a Travel Nurse Case Manager for ten years and have been all over the country.

Made in the USA
Lexington, KY
27 January 2019